Ethical Constraints and Imperatives in Medical Research

Publication Number 983
AMERICAN LECTURE SERIES®

A Monograph in
The BANNERSTONE DIVISION *of*
AMERICAN LECTURES IN BEHAVIORAL SCIENCE AND LAW

Edited by

RALPH SLOVENKO, B.E., LL.B., M.A., Ph.D.

Wayne State University
Law School
Detroit, Michigan

Ethical Constraints and Imperatives in Medical Research

By

MAURICE B. VISSCHER, Ph.D., M.D.

University of Minnesota Medical School
Minneapolis, Minnesota

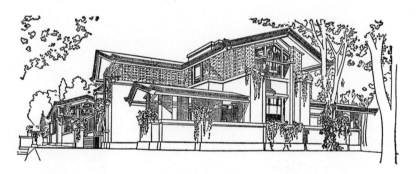

CHARLES C THOMAS · PUBLISHER
Springfield · Illinois · U.S.A.

Published and Distributed Throughout the World by
CHARLES C THOMAS • PUBLISHER
Bannerstone House
301-327 East Lawrence Avenue, Springfield, Illinois, U.S.A.

© *1975, by* CHARLES C THOMAS • PUBLISHER
ISBN 0-398-03404-4
Library of Congress Catalog Card Number: 74-32185

*With THOMAS BOOKS careful attention is given to all details of
manufacturing and design. It is the Publisher's desire to present books that are
satisfactory as to their physical qualities and artistic possibilities and
appropriate for their particular use. THOMAS BOOKS will be true to those
laws of quality that assure a good name and good will.*

Printed in the United States of America
C-1

Library of Congress Cataloging in Publication Data

Visscher, Maurice Bolks, 1901-
    Ethical constraints and imperatives in medical
research.

    (American lectures series; publication no. 983. A
monograph in the Bannerstone division of American lectures in behavioral science and law)
    Bibliography: p.
    Includes index.
    1. Human experimentation in medicine. 2. Medical
research—Moral and religious aspects. I. Title.
DNLM: 1. Ethics, Medical. 2. Human experimentation.
3. Research. W20.5 V833e
R853.H8V57   174'.2   74-32185
ISBN 0-398-03404-4

Preface

So many essays and books dealing with the ethics of biomedical research have been published in the past few years that an author must have good reasons for adding more to the literature. My reasons are several. First, too little attention has been paid to the wide range in the degrees of pertinence of various ethical considerations in the use of human subjects in scientific study. The vast difference has not been sufficiently emphasized between the ethical propriety of utilizing routine physical findings and laboratory data from patients with various diseases, in *ex post facto* studies of particular disease states, without going through the routine of obtaining "informed consent" from every subject source of laboratory or clinical data, and the propriety of failing to obtain such consent when some potentially injurious procedure is to be instituted in an experimental study.

Ethical considerations in relation to medical research ordinarily deal with a collection of prohibitions. "Thou shalt not . . ." do this or that is the usual form of treatment of the ethics of medical research. Too frequently the ethical imperative "Thou shalt . . ." do some positive act in promoting medical scientific advance is ignored. This book is written partly to point out explicitly that although ethical considerations do obviously impose constraints on actions, they equally impose imperatives for positive action in carrying on research. Hopefully this treatment will encourage a balanced view of the ethical problems for medical investigators and for the rest of society.

The scientific quest has an ethics of its own, and the implications of this built-in set of moral standards will be examined briefly.

Another reason for preparing this book is that the growing cult of "reverence for all life" is threatening the future of research employing lower animals, particularly cats and dogs because of their position as pets. The logic, or perhaps better the illogic, of the Albert Schweitzer philosophic position with respect to reverence for all life needs exposition and clarification if society is not to be harmed by the emotional biases of the zoophiles–who are frequently also anthropophobes–who are acquiring progressively greater influence. They are becoming more vocal and more influential all over the Western World, not simply in the United States. It is not without significance that as the kinship between man and other animals becomes clearer many people fail to recognize the obvious uniqueness of man in the animal hierarchy. Many modern humanists appear to have lost sight of the fact that there are orders of magnitude of difference in mental capacities between the human and any other surviving mammalian or other animal species in the world today. The zoophiles are impressed by their own anthropomorphic interpretations of animal behavior and psychology and attempt to have written into law their emotionally arrived at biases as to ethical principles in dealing with lower animals used as pets, particularly as to the intentional sacrifice of animals' lives in scientific study.

A further reason for this book is the fact that very poor logic has frequently been employed in dealing with such problems as the ethics of scientific research on specific groups of human subjects. Studies on children and on mental patients, for example, are frequently condemned, as is the use of prison inmates, totally ignoring the very real necessity for their own sakes to study many problems on children and mental patients, and the potential virtue to prison inmates to be allowed to participate of their own free will in socially useful projects. Another specific problem about which there is great emotional turmoil and consequent disagreement as to ethics is in the scientific use of the products of human conception after legal abortions. No area of medical research has stirred up so much turmoil in the United States as has the use of nonviable material from abortions, except perhaps the employment of beagle dogs in toxicity studies in medical research in Air Force and Army laboratories. The use of embryonic or fetal materials has involved religious controversies totally unrelated to the research programs themselves. The tremendous furor over DOD procurement authorization for thoroughbred beagles was made possible because it brought together on a single issue opponents of military expenditures, pacifists, pet lovers and antivivisectionists of all stripes.

The cooperative actions of various otherwise intellectually incompatible groups have created confusion over basic issues. An attempt has been made in this book to put the several issues into perspective in relation to more basic ethical considerations.

One cannot consider fully ethical problems of public interest without encountering the phenomenon of attempts to write into law the private moral prejudices of pressure groups of more or less political clout. Pressure politics, rather than ethics, is all too frequently the stimulus for legislative action in every area of social concern, and this is especially true in connection with the use of animals in scientific study. It would be a great mistake in considering ethical problems in medical research not to examine the unethical character of potentially powerful political lobbies opposing the use of particular lower animals in biomedical science studies. The same is true in connection with the use of nonviable human embryonic or fetal material.

Another reason for this book is the need to stress the basic factors responsible for the current increase in concern for the ethical problems in medical research. The first obvious factor is the huge increase in the magnitude of the enterprise over the last quarter century. A second is the fact that such research is now reaching into areas such as genetic engineering, "test-tube babies" and the like, where the emotionally charged results of research begin to appear on the horizon.

Because of the fact that most treatments of the subject of the ethics of medical research deal primarily with the prevention of potential evils which could possibly be perpetrated by investigators using human or animal subjects for scientific study, I shall point out that the use of both human and animal subjects under proper conditions is not only ethically justified but that we are under a moral imperative to carry out such studies in an ethical society. In other words, I intend to turn the argument around and ask whether it is not immoral to impose unnecessary impediments to medical research. There are two sides to every coin.

The author is grateful for the support of the Louis W. and Maud Hill Family Foundation in the preparation of this manuscript.

Contents

*Ethical Constraints
and Imperatives in
Medical Research*

CHAPTER 1

What Makes the Ethics of Medical Research a Pressing Problem?

E THICAL CONCERNS OF SOCIETY at any time are related to the contemporary human scene. Every age brings different ethical problems to the fore, and the late twentieth century is no exception. Among the newly crucial ethical problems today are those associated with the use of both human and animal subjects in biological–mainly medical–research. Ethical questions are arising today in the case of the employment of human subjects for investigative purposes, not because humans had not been subject to trial and error procedures in innovative medical practice in earlier times, but because with the rise of science and technology, in chemistry, physics and basic biomedical fields, research of a more sophisticated sort has become more possible and fruitful in the field of the clinical sciences.

It is primarily the phenomenal rise in basic scientific knowledge in the past century that has made clinical investigation productive and therefore more extensively pursued, rather than any recent change in the general ethical positions, either of the majority of physicians or the public, that has brought about the current interest in formulating definitive codes of ethics for clinical research.

Although science and technology have been evolving throughout human history, it is only in the last half or three quarters of a century that they have become controlling factors in all of our lives, whether we realize it or not, and whether we like it or not. Scientific advances have occurred on a logarithmic scale on a broad front. Increments in knowledge occur more rapidly the larger the base of knowledge on which additions can be built. Many other factors are partly responsible for the exponential rate of growth. Perhaps the most important is the fact that with every

3

new labor-saving discovery and invention, more and more people can be spared from the elemental tasks of growing food and building shelter and making gadgets, allowing them to spend their time and energies at science and creative technology, or other pursuits not immediately related to production and distribution of consumer goods and services. Consequently more men and women today than ever before in human history are devoting their working lives to scientific pursuits, including medical science.

The period between 1950 and 1968 was a golden age for medical science support, activity and accomplishment. It should be noted that from 1969 to 1974 there has been in the United States an official Federal administrative effort to stop growth in the medical research enterprise, except in relation to cancer and heart disease, in fact even to bring about cutbacks. Nevertheless the legislative bodies, which undoubtedly more closely reflect citizen-voter sentiment, have repeatedly at least partially frustrated those efforts to diminish overall investments in medical science progress. It is unlikely that the medical research enterprise will undergo eclipse, unless there is a worldwide catastrophic collapse of national economies.

Consequently one need not suppose that concern over the ethics of medical research will diminish. It will probably increase because with increased industrialization of underdeveloped countries there will be an overall increase in the scientific manpower of the world, with corresponding increases in attention paid to the social and ethical implications of science generally and medical science in particular.

A further reason for widespread human concern about the ethics of medical research is the blunt fact that in the name of research, ethical principles have in fact been violated in our lifetimes in too many instances. In what was falsely called medical research, atrocities were committed by Nazi physicians during the Hitler period. Exposure of these acts were directly responsible for the formulation of the Nuremburg and Helsinki declarations (see Appendices A and B) outlining proper ethical principles involved in acceptable use of human subjects in research. It must be noted that the German concentration camp atrocities were widely denounced by scientists and physicians around the world as soon as they became known. The shock and revulsion generated among physicians accomplished a very important result. It forced medical investigators to formulate more precisely the basic human rights of any persons used as subjects of medical or other scientific study. In other words, the demonstrated atrocities of the Nazi physicians involved in obvious criminal acts started a groundswell of interest in the whole field of ethics of human experimentation.

Furthermore, the more recent exposures of improprieties in the United States in connection with the so-called controlled late syphilis therapy study in Tuskogee which was continued far longer than was justified on any grounds, and the cancer cell injection studies in New York, as well as reports of coercion in studies of drug toxicity in prison systems such as in Arkansas, and other instances, have made people acutely aware of the fact that more safeguards must be set up in order to prevent abuses in the future.

As Chauncey Leake has documented in considerable detail in a recent essay,[1] from earliest times in all cultures the codes of conduct for physicians were humanistically oriented to the welfare of individual patients. The ethical physician and his helpers were to guard the rights and strive for benefits to patients as persons. The Hippocratic Oath, anachronistic as it may be in several regards, as in its prohibition against "cutting for stone," which was undoubtedly a reflection of the low regard at that time for barber-surgeons, was in its essentials a code of conduct which put the patient's interests first. To be sure it was also protective of the medical guild, but it was nevertheless a "consumer protection" statement. And today, despite the obvious failure of some few physicians to put the patient's welfare ahead of financial reward, the ethos of the profession at large is humanistic. The surgeon who advises and performs unnecessary surgery is not respected, although it must be admitted that guild protectiveness is one reason why such types of improprieties still occur. Physicians are in general loathe to criticize their confreres. This is true, however, primarily because medical practice is not an exact science, and most mistakes made by physicians are honest ones, due as much to the inherent uncertainties in diagnosis and in predictions as to the outcome of therapeutic procedures as to any other factor. Of course, ignorance of current knowledge is in itself a not inconsequential factor in producing low-grade medical practice.

There is some carryover of the attitude of reluctance of physicians to criticize their colleagues for malpractice in conventional health care into the field of research. This is certainly not universal, because physicians have been among the most bitter critics of clinical investigations of which they disapproved. Beecher,[2] for example, has excoriated some of his colleagues for infractions of those principles of ethical conduct in clinical research which he considers inviolate.

It has been the concern of members of the medical profession at least as much as the concern of laymen that has made the ethics of the employment of human subjects in medical research a currently important matter. It will undoubtedly always remain a lively subject because new real situations develop when such developments as discoveries in means of altering genetic material occur, just as new controversies arose when living human embryonic and fetal material became available when abortion was legalized in various countries. This is meant to be simply an example.

Ongoing ethical dialogue in connection with the employment of human subjects in scientific research is of great importance to humanity because men everywhere place high value on individual human rights, human dignity and compassion, and also place high value on improved health, longevity and social tranquility. Since neither external situations nor research possibilities are static, ethical judgments as to proprieties are bound to change. Continuing rational consideration of these problems will be part of social evolution.

REFERENCES

1. Leake, Chauncey: The humanistic tradition in the health professions. In Visscher, M. B. (Ed.): *Humanistic Perspectives in Medical Ethics.* Buffalo, Prometheus Books, 1973, Chap. 1, p. 7.
2. Beecher, H. K.: Ethics and clinical research. *N Eng J Med, 274:*1354-1360, 1966; and Beecher, H. K.: *Experimentation in Man.* Springfield, Thomas, 1959.

CHAPTER 2

Observations on the General Problem of Science and Ethics

SCIENTISTS AND LAYMEN as well have generally read too much into the truism that scientific facts are "amoral," and have paid too little attention to the equally obvious fact that scientists as persons are not exempt from ethical obligations. In recent years since science has become such a preponderant factor in every facet of human life, scientists themselves have begun to delve more deeply into the philosophic aspects of what might be called scientific ethics. In an essay entitled "From Biology to Ethics," the Nobel Laureate Jacques Monod[1] has recently suggested that a single ethic of devotion to objective truth will ordinarily take care of all the other problems. Perhaps if everyone were omniscient and could arrive at objective truth about all matters of human importance, such a point of view might be justified, because the human consequences would be among the elements of objective truth that would be essential to decision making. Bronowski[2] has elaborated similar views, and Bentley Glass[3] has extended these ideas, attempting to deduce the existence of ethical precepts within the scientific enterprise. They have emphasized complete truthfulness, fearlessness in defending unfettered scientific inquiry, and the necessity to communicate one's findings fully to the world as ethical imperatives. Obviously, such full communication would involve warnings to society of all of the consequences that might follow from the utilization and implementation of particular advances in scientific knowledge and in technology. The discussion of risks as well as benefits, and honest disclosure of uncertainties would certainly go far toward imposing a humanist ethic upon every scientist.

Jacques Monod stated categorically "science is ignorant of values," but he undoubtedly meant that it is only science in the abstract that is not concerned with morals, while the scientist in the

7

flesh cannot possibly escape from the problems of value judgments in behavior if he accepts the ethic of complete truthfulness.

It is certainly true that there is a built-in imperative to respect the truth in any scientific enterprise. No falsification of data nor distortion of interpretation can possibly survive in a system in which independently verifiable facts are its primary substance. Attempts at fraud have always eventually brought discredit to any scientist who was so stupid as to attempt to deceive.

Treatment of this topic would not be adequate without some explicit reference to instances in which scientists have failed the ethical imperative of honesty in the scientific method and philosophy. The prominent examples of dishonesty really only underscore the validity of the thesis that no professed scientist can long survive unless he or she does adhere to the principle of complete honesty. As Faber[4] has pointed out, "The emphasis on scientific success creates a severe strain on the practicing researcher, who is torn between the norms established for the process of research and the penultimate rewards for success. Under these conditions deviance is likely to occur in any group, even among scientists." Faber wrote in connection with the recent Summerlin falsifications at the Sloan-Kettering Institute for Cancer Research. Faber admits that attempts by others to confirm Summerlin's reports did bring about prompt exposure of this particular fraud, but he questions whether many lesser frauds do not remain undetected. It is true that "selection" of data, or even falsification of data do occur, but Faber has failed to recognize that the very existence of the competitiveness in science, and especially in the medical science field make it extremely probable that villains will be caught. If one wished one could cite a half dozen instances in this century in which fraud occurred and was promptly exposed. In one case a senior investigator committed suicide after the exposure because his assistant deceived him in his laboratory reports.

In a recent essay on what he calls "bioethics," Potter[5] has argued for the existence of some preexisting ethical imperatives that are peculiar to science. Potter has developed what he calls a "bioethical creed" to provide a practical code for individual behavior on the basis of a combination of biological knowledge and human values.

Of course, bioethics embraces larger areas than the ethics of medical research, but it encompasses the latter. Potter is greatly concerned, as are many biologists including the late Rachel Carson, Barry Commoner and Paul Erlich, among many others, with the perils of biological survival in the exhaustion of resources and the poisoning of the environment, as well as with the population explosion. These are problems of great medical importance, but other problems of medical importance also exist in the area of bioethics. One cannot deal with the science of genetics, for example, without considering fully the consequences to society of such currently interesting possible procedures as cloning or other entirely plausible major developments in human genetic engineering, without recognizing that their implementation would bring about great changes in society. The nature of those changes can perhaps only be hypothesized at the present time, but the ethic of truthfulness which is the foundationstone of science, requires that risks, benefits and uncertainties be fully disclosed. What Monod, Bronowski, Glass and Potter, among others, are arguing is that the central ethic of science, without which it could not exist, is itself a basis for the ethical imperatives which should and must control the behavior of scientists if either science or society is to survive. It is in this basic context that the ethics of medical research should and must be considered.

Anyone who considers problems of morality thoughtfully must confront the basic question of the kind of foundation one can give to the arguments that are raised. For centuries philosophers have been in a quandary as to how to justify fundamental principles of morality. There is a current urgency to a better understanding of the basis of human ethics, which was much less acute in the prescientific era than it is today. The rise of science has done two things simultaneously. It has multiplied by a large factor the capacity of immoral men to do damage, even to the extent of destroying all life, and it has loosened the underpinnings of the ethics of authoritarianism revealed in religions. Herbert Feigl[6] put the question, "In our age of scientific enlightenment we often ask ourselves what kind of foundation we can give to morality, to our basic commitments, to human rights and human equality? This is, of course, not an easy question to answer. It seems to some people much more convenient to appeal to transempirical authority. Often the question is raised, 'What lends authority to the ethical principles without which we could not survive?' I believe that the cynicism and anarchism we see in so many young people today represents a danger not only for the survival of civilization and for human well-being, but even for the psychological well-being of the individual concerned. Now what can we say in this connection?"

Feigl is pessimistic about achieving a consensus about any moral question without a prior consensus about some basic objectives for moral behavior. On this score he has said, "I am quite inclined to say that you won't get any place with ethical justification unless you start with certain commitments. The adoption of those commitments can be made palatable, but there is nothing that we can prove or disprove about them. To be sure, utilitarians and hedonists try to show that if we are to have the greatest happiness for the greatest number, then these moral precepts commend themselves for adoption; but of course this idea presupposes already that the major aim, the greatest good of the greatest number, is itself morally desirable." In this view his opinion is not unlike that of A. J. Ayer,[7] who wrote, "We find that argument is possible on moral questions only if some system of values is presupposed."

Nevertheless we are certainly under great compulsion to find generally acceptable grounds for defining what is good and arranging societal affairs in such ways that human behavior will approach more generally as closely as possible to what it ought to be in order to achieve that good.

In the life and work of the physician there has been since ancient times the presupposition that human values are paramount. Thus there has been a basic principle from which logical processes can begin. The real situation is therefore more distressful to the professional logician than it is to the physician, or indeed to men generally. As a philosopher, Feigl is obviously unhappy about the lack of an easy logic in relation to human values and moral ideals. He has said, "So I think that a unified set of supreme moral values can be empirically discerned as inherent in the conscience of man, even if it is not always displayed in his behavior. We cannot, how-ever, get away from the fact that human needs and interests and human nature in general are highly relevant for human values or moral ideals. I assume a sort of synthesis between a 'nothing but' and a 'something more' view of morality; namely, morality on the one hand is relative to human interests, and moral values neither come down from on high nor are dictated by the deity. There is a golden mean that combines the valid element of monism, i.e. that ethical principles are universally applicable, with the empiricism of relativism which teaches that human values are related to human nature. If you want a label for this call it 'scientific humanism.' "

In considering ethical problems in medical research on human subjects one must be mindful of the deceptiveness of the apparently simple maxim "the greatest good for the greatest number," because in specific cases damage to the interest of one individual may outweigh the potential advantage to a very large number of individuals. In fact, the kernel of the problem in achieving agreement about the ethics of human experimentation lies in the search for guidelines for harmonizing the desire for universally applicable principles with the need for recognition that every situation is in reality different from any other.

REFERENCES

1. Monod, Jacques: *From Biology to Ethics,* trans. by Keith Botsford. Lecon inaugurale, College de France, 1967.
2. Bronowski, Jr.: *Science and Human Values.* NYC, Messner, 1956.
3. Glass, Bentley: *Science and Ethical Values.* Chapel Hill, N.C., University of Carolina Press, 1965; and The ethics of science. *Science, 150:*1254, 1965.
4. Faber, Bernard L.: The Sloan-Kettering affair. *Letters in Science, 185 (4153):*734, 1974.
5. Potter, Van R.: Social ethics and the conduct of science. *Annals of New York Academy of Science,* December 1971.
6. Feigl, Herbert: In Kurtz, Paul (Ed.): *Problems of Morality in Our Age of Science.* Buffalo, Prometheus Press, 1970.
7. Ayer, A. J.: In Barrett, W., and Aiken, H. D. (Eds.): *Philosophy in the Twentieth Century.* New York, Random House, 1962, Vol. 3, pp. 87-101.

CHAPTER 3

Medical Research on Human Subjects as a Moral Imperative

Primum non nocere

THE USE OF HUMAN SUBJECTS in biomedical research is considered by scientists to be indispensible to progress in medical science and to consequent improvement in the art of medical practice, but the protection of the rights and welfare of every human being is equally a first priority of a civilized society. So long as these two basic precepts are not in conflict there are no major ethical problems in connection with scientific study on human subjects. However, there are situations in which the two objectives can clash, and then ethical problems arise.

In the practice of medicine the classic principle *primum non nocere* could be, if one knew what might be harmful, a simple rule to follow. Unfortunately even in ordinary medical practice such certainty is impossible. Intentional harm can be avoided, but unintentional harm cannot yet be avoided because of lack of adequate knowledge of human biology, broadly defined. Thus one comes, in attempting to fulfill the primary obligation of the medical profession, "first do no harm," to an ethical imperative to the profession as a whole and to the investigative physician specifically to make studies to learn how to avoid doing harm to patients. In other words, physicians frequently cannot properly perform their first function fully unless more research is done. This may be, to some, a different twist to the problem of ethics of medical practice, including the investigative use of human subjects, from the more simplistic views of the past. If it is, as seems obvious, obligatory upon physicians to learn how to do no harm, then scientific investigation, including that on human subjects becomes a necessity for an ethical medical profession. Equally it becomes an activity which society at large must, if it wishes to provide a milieu in which medicine can be practiced ethically, promote the conditions under which medical and related research can be carried out in harmony with humanistic ethics.

The learned pharmacologist, Nobel Laureate Professor B. N. Halpern,[1] who discovered and developed numerous widely used and important new therapeutic agents, has stated the case very convincingly. In a recent essay he wrote in connection with studies of drug toxicity and effectiveness.

> I should like to stress yet again most forcefully that, in the interests of science and even of the protection of society against the absolutely unpredictable collective damage that the introduction of a new drug may cause, it is indispensable that trials in man should be included in pharmacological research.
>
> The term "human experimentation" raises a sinister echo in each of us, for reasons known to us all. But fear solves no scientific problems. For my part, the recommendations . . . that safety tests of new drugs should be carried out on fully informed volunteers in conditions of almost absolute security—is more in conformity with the requirements of ethics than the thousands of such trials hypocritically carried out daily in hospitals in all countries on individuals who are totally ignorant of what is being done to them.

Writing on the topic, "Justification for the Human Trial," Beecher[2] has said,

> The importance of the project undertaken must be commensurate with the risk involved. The insurance of this is a cardinal responsibility of all who undertake experimentation in man. But having stated that important principle, there is still a vast area where judgment—one hopes sound judgment—must operate. Only the fanatic denies that animal experimentation must precede the human. As Sir Geoffrey Jefferson put it, "Man is too rare, too expensive, altogether too valuable an animal" to be first used in study of technical procedures or trial of even therapeutic agents. There are (nevertheless) species differences. Ultimately, the definitive test must be done in man.

This is obviously true because, although certain similarities are found in fundamental processes from the simplest organisms to man, as in the general mechanisms of information storage in the genetic apparatus, and in the basic building blocs of certain enzymes, there are also very important differences between species, becoming greater the farther they are apart in the phylogenetic tree. Even within a single genus the possibilities for variations in gene combinations are so great that aside from single ovum twins or the products of many generations of inbreeding important differences between individuals are evident in many characteristics. Histoincompatibility as a cause of the usual homograft rejection is evidence that even at the molecular level individuality is the rule. Fortunately for the applicability of blood transfusion in therapy, the existence as first discovered by Landsteiner, of major blood types, within which differences in properties of agglutinins for red blood cells are ordinarily so small as to permit survival of the cells. An extension of Landsteiner's discovery, and others based upon it, into the field of tissue and organ transplantation is also yielding promising results.

It is, of course, not only in the area of immunology that individuality is important. Reactions to drugs of all sorts differ, not only in different species but among individuals of a single species or even a single genus. For example, the doses of digitalis glycosides required to produce a given effect in a rat are orders of magnitude higher than those needed per unit body weight in a cat or a man. Some drug effects seen in one species, or even in an entire family within a particular class, are not seen at all in another class. It is partly for these reasons that drug studies must be carried out in many species of lower animals before even planning to use them in man. And because of the intraspecies, and intragenus variability of individuals one must eventually study the effects of new agents on large numbers of humans in order to know what the limiting parameters for both efficacy and safety are. Furthermore the physician must know how to assess the idiosyncracies of individual patients in their responsiveness to pharmaceutical agents, and must understand as much as is known about the principles of action of such agents if he is to be a reliable physician.

There is also a need to study human subjects in connection with disease entities which are unique to man, or almost so. Likewise with respect to nervous and mental processes, although much can be learned by studies on lower animals, particularly with respect to basic neural mechanisms, there remain those features of function that are uniquely human which would forever remain shrouded in mystery if the scientific method were not to be employed to throw light upon them.

In other words, it is a fanciful dream concocted in the minds of scientific illiterates that medical science, or any other biological science, could progress without the study of actual living systems, and ultimately in the case of medicine, study of living human subjects.

There is a corollary to these lines of reasoning. It is that there is an ethical imperative for physicians as a group to promote medical research, including studies on human subjects. Obviously for various reasons not every physician can be an investigator, but at least every physician should give moral support to the enterprise of advancement of medical knowledge. The vast majority of physicians accept this view in principle, but in practice many fail to act to promote the medical research enterprise.

The conclusions of Claude Bernard[3] in his *Introduction to the Study of Experimental Medicine,* written a little more than a century ago are undoubtedly pertinent today. He said, "For we must not deceive ourselves, morals do not forbid making experiments on one's neighbor or on one's self; in everyday life men do nothing but experiment on one another. Christian morals forbid only one thing, doing ill to one's neighbor. So, among the experiments that may be tried on man, those that can only harm are forbidden, those that are innocent are permissible, and those that may do good are obligatory."

REFERENCES

1. Halpern, B. N.: CIOMS round tables: 1. *Biomedical Science and the Dilemma of Human Experimentation.* Paris, UNESCO House, 1967, pp. 30 and 31.
2. Beecher, Henry K.: *Experimentation in Man.* Springfield, Thomas, 1958, p. 32.
3. Bernard, Claude as translated by Henry Copley Greene: *An Introduction to the Study of Experimental Medicine.* U.S.A., Henry Schuman, 1927, p. 102.

CHAPTER 4

The Ethics of the Use of
Human Subjects in Research
in Relation to Its Legal Control

PERSONAL ETHICS are the rules one chooses to live by. *Laws* are the rules the state attempts to force people to live by. Ideally, the two might be the same, but of course in reality they frequently are not. Laws are written primarily in response to political pressures, and not solely as a result of deliberative analysis of objective facts. It is interesting that the adjectives "ethical" and "legalistic" have such widely different connotations. It is because the two concepts are so far apart that one must deal with ethics and the law separately regardless of how much one might wish that the two were closer together. With respect to medical research, emotional factors have played a very great role in generating political pressure and in the passage of applicable law.

Medical research involves the use both of experimental animals and of human subjects, and both ethical and legal considerations are quite different in the two categories of methods of investigation. The interrelations of ethics and law for the two types of subjects of study must be considered somewhat separately. It should be noted that for the most part investigations aiming at basic biological principles can be studied more appropriately in lower forms of life than in man. This is because biological scientists view the sacrifice of life of lower forms of life very differently than they do the exposure of human subjects to risk of bodily or other injury.

Until recently, that is until roughly the last half century, clinical investigation involving the use of human subjects has ordinarily been closely tied to therapeutic procedures in medicine. There have, of course, been rare instances in which controlled experiments aimed at elucidating the etiology of disease, such as those performed on volunteers to investigate the means of transmission

16

of yellow fever were carried on. But the infrequency of such types of study in practice prevented giving rise to public concern. Furthermore, when physicians employed new drugs or surgeons utilized new and previously untried procedures in the treatment of patients, public concern was at a minimum because of two factors: First, the difficulty of distinguishing between the prerogatives of the physician in exercising professional judgment as to the methods of treatment that should be recommended, and second, the fact that there were no large organized clinical research facilities in operation. It has only been since, in the more advanced industrial societies, relatively large funds have been available for research involving the use of human subjects that the public and, by consequence, legislative bodies have concerned themselves with the problems in a forceful way.

Since most scientific medical studies using human subjects have been performed by physicians, the medical practice acts in various states in the United States have in the past provided a framework under which legal redress could be sought for wrongs committed or alleged to have been committed by investigative physicians. In a recent statement by Bernard Hirsh,[1] the General Counsel of the American Medical Association, the present situation has been summarized as follows, "Although the courts have not yet had the opportunity to develop special rules for determining the legal rights of individuals involved in clinical investigation, there are general rules of law that undoubtedly would be applied if litigation arises. The most significant of these general rules relate to compensation for medical malpractice and personal injury."

However, medical malpractice and personal injury suits deal only with compensation or with possible loss of licensure "after the fact." Regulatory law governing the use of human subjects "before the fact" is a very different approach. Legislative bodies have developed the regulatory approach to the solution of many problems in recent years. Regulations of executive departments, which have the force of law, are now common mechanisms for exercise of delegated authority. This is the mechanism that is now being developed to prevent abuses in connection with the employment of human subjects in medical research.

The United States Congress passed and the President signed

into law on July 13, 1974, the National Research Act which provides for the setting up of a Commission for the Protection of Human Subjects of Biomedical and Behavioral Research. Its Title II may be summarized as follows: The Secretary of Health, Education, and Welfare is to appoint the eleven members of the Commission. No more than five members may be persons who have been engaged in biomedical or behavioral research involving human subjects. The Secretary is charged with appointing individuals distinguished in the fields of medicine as well as law, ethics, theology, philosophy, humanities, health administration, government, and public affairs, and in the biological, physical, and behavioral sciences. The Commission is to be appointed within two months of the signing of the Act and is to complete its work not later than two years after its inception. It is to make periodic progress reports and a final report to the President, the Congress, and the Secretary within three months after the expiration of the two-year period.

The Commission is instructed first to conduct a comprehensive investigation to identify basic ethical principles which should underlie the conduct of biomedical and behavioral research involving humans. It is to develop guidelines for the conduct of such research in accordance with the principles identified above. The Commission is instructed to consider at least the following issues:

1. The boundaries between biomedical and behavioral research and the accepted routine practice of medicine.
2. The place of risk-benefit criteria in determining appropriateness of research.
3. Guidelines for the selection of subjects.
4. Nature and definition of informed consent in various situations.
5. Evaluating, monitoring, and enforcement mechanisms for the Institutional Review Boards now required by the Department of HEW.
6. Consideration of the appropriateness of applying guidelines to HEW health service programs.

It is to make recommendations to the Secretary for proper administrative action for the protection of subjects, as well as to identify informed consent requirements for research involving children, prisoners, and the mentally infirm. It is to investigate the need for a mechanism to assure protection for subjects not now subject to regulation by the Secretary of HEW. It is to investigate the nature and extent of research involving human fetuses, the purposes for which such research has been undertaken, and alternative means for achieving such purposes. This report shall make recommendations to the Secretary concerning conduct of such research within four months of the inception of the Commission. Until the Commission has made such recommendations, the Secretary is instructed not to "conduct or support research in the United States or abroad on a living fetus, before or after induced abortion of such fetus, unless such research is done for the purpose of assuring survival of such fetus." This is the only definitive prohibition in the Act.

The Commission is instructed to study the use of psychosurgery in the United States during the five-year period ending December 31, 1972. The Committee is to make recommendations to the Secretary concerning a policy for appropriate use (if any) of psychosurgery. It is also to study the ethical, social, and legal implications of advances in biomedical and behavioral research and technology.

Within two months of the receipt of any recommendation, the Secretary shall publish it in the *Federal Register* and elicit public comment. Within six months of publication, the Secretary shall publish a determination concerning the recommendation and the reasons for such determination.

After the Commission ceases to exist, there is to be established a permanent National Advisory Council for Protection of Subjects of Biomedical and Behavioral Research. The Council is to be appointed by the Secretary, composed of seven to fifteen members who have the same qualifications as the Commission. No member of the Commission will be eligible for appointment to the permanent Council. The Council is to make recommendations to the Secretary, review policies and regulations, and disseminate appropriate information to the public.

The Secretary shall require applicants for a grant or contract to submit satisfactory assurances to him that they have established Institutional Review Boards to review research involving humans conducted or sponsored by the applicants. He shall establish a program within the Department of HEW for clarification and guidance with respect to ethical issues raised in connection with research involving human subjects.

This Act represents the culmination of years of controversy within the Congress and in the public at large as to what legal mechanisms should be set up to monitor and regulate the use of human subjects in research. In its enacted form it recognizes that the Congress is not the body to set up the principles on which the propriety of particular types of research on human subjects should be judged, except, as noted, that in the case of research on human fetal material, the Congress bowed to the force of minority pressure groups and temporarily outlawed such research. However, in general the Act puts responsibility on a Commission and ultimately on a permanent Council to deal with this very important and controversial issue. If the members of the Commission and the Council are wisely chosen the result might be felicitous. If not, there could be catastrophic effects upon the progress of medical science and, through it, on medical practice. Only time will tell. At least the Act does not itself permanently proscribe any particular types of research and leaves the field open for rational discussions and decisions in the future.

The National Research Act of 1974, Title II, is a far cry from the many unwise proposals that have been made in the past. In recent years many Congressional bills have been introduced, some good, some very bad, and the present Act involved many compromises.

From an historical viewpoint it is of interest to note the U.S. Congressional interest in human experimentation has a three-quarter century history. On March 2, 1900 Senator Jacob Gallinger introduced a bill into the 1st Session of the 56th Congress bearing the number S. 3424. The title of the bill was "For the Regulation of Scientific Experiments on Human Beings in the District of Columbia." Senator Gallinger had been by profession a homeopathic physician, and was quite obviously totally unsympathetic with clinical investigation. The first section in the bill that he introduced reads as follows:

Be it enacted by the Senate and House of Representatives of the United States of America in Congress assembled, that no physician, surgeon, pathologist, student of medicine or of science, or any other person shall make or perform upon the body of any human being, in any hospital, asylum, retreat, or infirmary established for the treatment of the sick, or in any other place in the District of Columbia, any scientific experiment involving pain, distress, or risk to life and health, whether by administration of poisonous drugs for the purpose of ascertaining their toxicity, by inoculating the germs of disease, by grafting cancerous tumors into healthy tissues, or by performance of any surgical operation for any other object than the amelioration of the patient, except subject to the restrictions and regulations hereinafter prescribed. Any person performing, advising, or assisting in the performance of any such experiment upon any newborn babe, pregnant woman, lunatic, idiot, or patient, in any public or private hospital, in any infant's home, hospital asylum, or private house, or upon any other person whatsoever, shall be deemed guilty of the crime of human vivisection, and upon conviction shall be liable to a fine of not less than one thousand dollars or imprisonment for not less than one year, or both. If any such experiment shall be followed within forty-eight hours by the death of the person thus operated upon, or if it shall appear that death was accelerated in any way by such experiment, the performance of any such experiment shall be deemed manslaughter or murder, as the circumstances of the case shall determine; and all persons taking part therein shall be liable to the penalties prescribed for such crime.

It is of interest to note the severity of the penalties that Senator Gallinger proposed, some of which are reminiscent of the eye for an eye, and a life for a life type of penalty imposed for malpractice in very ancient times as described by Chauncey Leake.[2] However, it should be noted that in another section of the Gallinger bill he provided for exemption from its provisions, studies in which voluntary consent of subjects had been obtained and a special court order had been issued permitting the studies, so long as the subjects were not "under twenty years of age, pregnant, aged, infirm, epileptic, insane or feebleminded." The importance of the consent of subjects and the competence of the subject to understand what he or she was consenting to was evident in Gallinger's thinking. By implication too the "rights" of the unborn fetus were recognized in the exclusion of pregnant women from the category of permissible sane adults who could give consent.

The virtue in the 1974 Act, as compared with the abortive Gallinger 1900 Bill and others, is of course that the Congress itself
has not attempted to write the specifics with the exception, as
noted before, of studies on fetuses. There is evidence of much
greater sophistication in the current law. There is much advantage
in control by departmental regulation as opposed to statutory law
dealing with the intricacies of this problem. In the first place, although departmental regulations are obviously drawn up by legal
counsel, this is done with the detailed advice of persons who are
knowledgeable with regard to the actualities of problems in connection with the employment of human subjects in research. Now
the new Commission will undoubtedly have a controlling voice.
Statutory law is ordinarily drawn up in final form instead in executive sessions of Committees of the Congress and frequently reflect special interest political decisions without informed input. Till
now, at least, Congressional committees have lacked scientific staff
support. The executive departments are one step removed from
ordinary political pressures. Perhaps most important is the fact
that departmental regulations can be altered from time to time as
defects of one sort or another appear in prior stipulations. Assuming that the executive departments are genuinely concerned with
the proper protection of human subjects, which can be said to be
a fair assumption, it would appear that such a mechanism would
be far superior to any in which the details of the controlling rules
were "carved in stone," as they would be in Congressional Acts
which when once passed are very difficult to amend.

The need for assurance to the public today that the whims of
individual investigators who may sacrifice ethical propriety to sel-
fish interests is quite clear. In an essay on human experimentation the legal scholar Guido Calabresi[3] has written:

> We are committed to "humanism," to the dignity of the individ-
> ual, and to human life. Much of the fabric of our society depends on
> our belief in this commitment, as do most of our traditional and
> "cherished" liberties. Accident law indicates that our commitment to
> human life is not, in fact, so great as we say it is; that our commit-
> ment to life-destroying material progress and comfort is greater. But
> this fact merely accentuates our need to make a bow in the direction
> of our commitment to the sanctity of human life (whenever we can
> do so at a reasonable total cost). It also accentuates our need to re-

ject any societal decisions that too blatantly contradict this commitment. Like "free will," it may be less important that this commitment be total than that we believe it to be there.

The impression should not be given that no legal control over the use of human subjects in scientific study existed before the Act of 1974. Actually the Department of HEW and its National Institutes of Health have for a number of years acted to regulate human experimentation on their general authority to set up conditions for grants and contracts. In brief, control was and will still largely be exercised through a mandatory peer review mechanism by requiring institutions receiving funds for work involving the use of human subjects to set up an elaborate committee structure to control such work. However, the DHEW itself reserves the right to make judgments internally with respect to the adequacy of institutional committee control. Rules and regulations for the protection of human subjects have been revised from time to time but those currently in force have been issued in the name of the Department of Health, Education, and Welfare, and were published in the *Federal Register* for May 30, 1974. They are reproduced in part in Appendix C.

It should be recognized by all students of the problem that there are both virtues and hazards in the legal regulation of scientific studies on human subjects. The virtues are that both investigatees and investigators derive protection. The first from any recognizable improprieties and the second from unjustified criticism, and, if laws were to be properly framed, there could be protection against legal or economic penalties for mishaps to subjects treated according to approved study designs. There are obviously some legitimate and necessary types of clinical investigation in which there are some risks to the well-being of the subject. If the sanction for performance of such studies is granted on the basis of legally approved mechanisms, the investigator is more readily absolved from blame for any unfortunate consequences than he would be if no such legal sanction existed. Not only is the hazard of malpractice suits diminished, but it has been seriously proposed that a mechanism be set up on a national basis which would provide compensation to victims of such accidents or to their surviving dependents, if there are such. The justifiability of such a suggestion derives from the fact that society as a whole has much to gain by some types of potentially hazardous studies, for example, the first use on the human of newly developed vaccines against crippling diseases. It is a matter of record that some of the early recipients of poliomyelitis vaccines were crippled for life and some died. However, few people, if any, would maintain that the virtual conquest of poliomyelitis as an epidemic disease has not brought overwhelming societal benefits that are worth the cost. Nevertheless the harm done to a few individuals cannot be denied and should not be neglected.

The hazards exist in the fallibility of human judgment on the part of the peer review committees and in the difficulties in writing either statutory law or regulations in such a way as to cover all contingencies properly. Flexibility is a necessary ingredient in the administration of laws or of regulations which have the force of law. In any human situation in which there are multiple laudable and important human values at stake, it is likely that one good will conflict with another. This is the case in connection with current problems in the field of human experimentation. At several institutions in which large programs of biomedical research in a wide spectrum of fields are carried on, the committees charged with implementing current Federal policy have come up with internal regulations which, if maintained, cannot avoid grave damage to society. The Department of HEW regulations[4] properly place great emphasis on "informed consent." However, the protection of persons from psychological, social, and legal risks are nearly as heavily stressed as is protection against bodily harm. The applicable definitions of subjects at risk include "any individual who may be exposed to the possibility of psychological, or social injury, as a consequence of participation as a subject in any research, development, or related activity which departs from the application of those established and accepted methods necessary to meet his needs, or which increased the ordinary risks of daily life, including the recognized risks inherent in a chosen occupation or field of service." Psychological or social injuries are usually difficult and frequently impossible to define.

Whenever legislation or bureaucratic regulations for a general purpose are formulated there is a temptation to cover every possible exigency by statute or rule. In connection with the problem of research dealing with human subjects the territory that can be covered is so vast that one can envision great harm done to society in the name of protecting it. Take for example the admittedly important matter of protection of the right to privacy.

When an investigative physician writes up a case report, or a compilation of data on numerous patients whom he has treated in various ways, there is always a possibility that by some accident or even by some unlawful sleuthing by an ambitious newspaper or other media reporter, the identity of the subjects treated might become known. Much valuable information–important to human welfare–has been derived from *ex post facto* studies of patient data. Moreover, strictly speaking, such studies constitute the use of human subjects in scientific research and as such fall under the control of laws regulating such activity. And furthermore, personal privacy can possibly be invaded in such studies and reports. For example, when dealing with venereal disease or psychotropic drug use, grave harm to individuals could result from disclosure. Even the fact that an individual had been treated by a psychiatrist can be a matter of national political importance, and devastating to an individual, as recent United States political history has shown. In other words, concern about the rights of privacy is not a trivial matter.

However, to subject studies of clinical results of conventional or common forms of treatment to the rules governing human experimentation, including fully informed consent of every patient involved, seems to be carrying a principle to the absurd. No medical scientist identifies the patients about whom he writes because it is contrary to basic medical ethics. Later disclosure of identity of subjects is also very rare, except in spectacular research such as an organ transplantation. It is then usually the fault of some nosey reporter. He or she, not the investigator, should be made responsible for the harm, if any, done to the subject of a report.

In a different but equally important category are reports of studies made on urine, feces, or blood of patients, collected for diagnostic purposes, but studied in addition for other characteristics which are of interest to an investigator for one reason or another. The reason might be simply a statistical survey of the incidence of some disease or abnormality in a particular population. Or it might be an exploratory study of the correlation of one or another factor with the disease from which a patient is suffering. Or it might be a study of the incidence of some antigen or immune body in the general population.

How much, if anything, need the subject be told about the rationale of such studies, and need the investigator obtain informed consent in order for such a study to be ethical? The common-sense answers would seem to be that so long as the materials employed for study are simply ordinary clinical data or information gained from excess material from clinically indicated laboratory tests, the investigator has no obligation whatever to obtain consent from the subjects, so long as the anonymity of the subjects is protected.

But someone is sure to raise the question of whether the situation is not different when the clinically required laboratory data would require only one or two milliliters of blood, and the additional studies would utilize some excess which would otherwise be discarded. Would it not constitute, technically and legally, an "assault" to utilize the extra blood for another purpose? In practice one does not ordinarily draw the precise minimum amount of blood for particular laboratory tests for diagnostic purposes. Consequently in many instances no really valid question arises although present rules would require informed consent.

However in instances in which relatively large quantities of blood are needed for a research study, the researcher certainly has an obligation to obtain informed consent. The common-sense answer to the problem would seem to be that informed consent should be required only when significant quantities of blood, over and above those necessary for indicated clinical diagnostic purposes, are required for a study.

These points are raised because there will certainly be controversies in the future about such problems unless in both statutes and administrative regulations some common-sense distinctions are always made between investigative procedures which pose actual hazards to human subjects and those that do not. This is perhaps most frequently important when the only possible theoretical hazard is invasion of privacy.

Since invasion of privacy is an important offense in certain types of situation it would appear that one should distinguish between protecting it, and the need to explain the purposes, and the hazards if they exist, which they do not in the instances cited, of the scientific study. Safeguarding privacy is certainly justified in all instances, but informed consent as to totally innocuous procedures appears to be superfluous, especially when the procedures are performed on urine, feces and blood collected for clinically indicated purposes.

The same line of reasoning applies to *ex post facto* analyses of the relative merits of conventional types of therapy. However, a very different situation arises when prospective studies of new drugs or procedures are involved. In this situation definite risk factors are frequently involved and informed consent becomes relevant and obligatory on ethical grounds.

Special mention should be made of the problems now arising in retrospective population studies of the incidence of certain types of disease. At the present time, epidemiologists at the University of California in Los Angeles, carrying out questionnaire studies of the incidences of a wide variety of neurological diseases, are being forced to obtain informed consent from thousands of prospective interviewees, before they may ask them a single question. The absurdity of that requirement is evident, first from the fact that fully informing the subject requires explaining all of the proposed questions, and second—even more important—is that the interviewee can withdraw from participation in the interview at any time, even after having answered all the questions, or any fraction of them. Even granting the possibility that recalling and recounting one's personal and family medical history may be an anxiety-raising experience, it seems absurd to require the facade of obtaining a signed consent form before asking a question and requiring at the same time that all of the questions to be asked be explained before the interviewee can be asked to sign a document which he or she can later withdraw. Epidemiological research can be hampered and the public welfare hurt unless such rules are modified.

At another institution, the Columbia-Presbyterian Medical Center,[5] the institution has ruled that investigators may not, without obtaining informed consent, use blood, sweat, urine and feces for any investigative purpose, even if the material had been collected initially for diagnostic purposes. Likewise at the University of Minnesota[6] a similar prohibition is outlined. The precise wording of the Institutional Committee regulation with regard to this problem is as follows:

Collection of Data for Beneficial Services Distinguished from Research Involving SUBJECTS Using Such Data.

In a number of situations within the University or where procedures are performed under the auspices of the University, diagnostic or therapeutic procedures of benefit to the individual upon whom they are performed or conducted in the provision of professional services may be undertaken with the foreknowledge that the record of such procedures or services or the products of such procedures or services will ultimately be the subject of future study and evaluation which would constitute "research involving human subjects" within the meaning given that phrase in this policy. Where the procedures or performance of services would be undertaken normally and be the type of professional service for the direct benefit of the individual subject to the procedures, rather than for purpose of obtaining information for advancement of human knowledge, the original performance of such procedures or professional services will not constitute "research involving human subjects" or "procedures involving human subjects" as those terms are used in this Statement of Policy.

However, the subsequent use of the records or products of such professional services for purposes other than the direct benefit of the subject or someone related to him or her or for other than clinical training and primarily for the advancement of knowledge that shall be considered to be "research involving human subjects" and the present policy and any procedures designed for its furtherance in the safeguarding of rights and welfare of human subjects shall be applicable to this subsequent use of record data.

It should be noted that the same prohibitions apply to the use of material derived from a biopsy or an autopsy. In fact, of course, no autopsy is ever performed except by coroners looking for evidence of foul play, unless one hopes to gain some new scientific information. This is obviously research. It is true that permission from next of kin is necessary to make an autopsy legal, but the content of permission forms is not such as to constitute informed consent.

Many institutions maintain banks of biomedically useful materials. Blood banks are an example. Strict interpretation of rules would make it improper to utilize information concerning blood types, antibody titers, and any other scientific information concerning samples of banked blood for any research study without individual informed consent. Hundreds, perhaps thousands, of such studies have already been reported in the past. In no case has informed consent been obtained from the donors, although legal permission to obtain the blood and waivers of responsibility for accidents may have been.

The unreality of the implications of some of the Federal guidelines and the rigid interpretations placed upon them by cautious institutional authorities must be apparent to anyone considering the problem objectively. The institutions that set up rigid rules may only be attempting to call attention to some of the absurdities in the situation, but more likely they are attempting to demonstrate, on paper at least, that they are like Caesar's wife, above suspicion.

It is the public that will be hurt unless paranoid fears of invasion of privacy are allayed in some other manner than by the imposition of rigid informed consent rules for stored clinical data or biological materials. This is particularly true because in many instances deep-freeze banks of material are maintained for years without any prior determination as to what information it might be decided at a later date could be obtained from such samples. The donors may be dead or have moved to another location and their addresses be unknown. Should potential sources of information be closed because of the practical impossibility of obtaining informed consent? This is one of the questions that society at large will have to answer.

If some legal mechanism for protecting privacy in such situations seems desirable, let it be one which imposes penalties on the individuals who are responsible for the important aspects of invasion of privacy, namely those who disclose the identity of individuals, materials from whom have been studied. It is a virtual certainty that no serious medical scientist will be penalized by such a rule. A prying reporter interested in scandal might be exposed to some legal hazards if he or she disclosed improperly obtained information, but this is quite another problem.

The ethical problem is simply one of whether a hypothetical good can possibly be given determining weight in the total ethical equation when adherence to rules protecting against its possible infraction make impossible the achievement of a genuine good of great importance to human welfare. One deals with a total situation in practical ethical judgments. When there are competing goods it would seem obvious that the genuine should outweigh the hypothetical.

There is a real danger today that the burdensomeness of methods involved with forestalling largely or completely imaginary hazards to human subjects which are being imposed on investigators may greatly impede legitimate and humanly valuable and important research. One can concede and even insist that there is a need today for effective restraints upon some types of human investigation and yet insist equally strongly that other types of restraints are both unnecessary and undesirable.

There is a specific type of objection on the part of some "protectionist" groups today to which reference should be made, because it is so important to the future of clinical investigation. There is objection to the employment of procedures for randomizing the selection of subjects for particular forms of treatment in which comparisons are to be made of the effectiveness of one or another procedure. A case in point is a study funded with Federal funds being carried on in a number of institutions in which three currently conventional methods of surgical management of cancer of the breast are being compared. Each method is in wide use by competent surgeons and no one knows whether or not there is a particular virtue in any one. This is explained to the patients, who are fully informed and have agreed to the randomization method, which is simply the chance selection of one card in three after the establishment of a diagnosis following biopsy. However, the complaint is being made by critics that the subjects may not realize that randomization means selection by pure chance, which is being condemned. It happens that in the particular instance cited the results show no superiority in any of the three methods of surgical management which involve in the three protocols progressively more radical dissection of underlying structures in the second and third protocols as compared with the first. There is no way in which the information obtained could have been gained without comparison of results in a totally randomized study, because if the surgeon were to decide in each case what operation to perform, he or she would be inclined to advocate the more drastic procedure in cases in which there seemed to be more urgent indications.

The objection being made to the practice of randomization of management designation has broad implications because no valid comparison of effectiveness, not only of surgical procedures, but of drug therapy can be made without such a study. There are many current controversies as to the superiority or inferiority of widely accepted types of drug therapy for various illnesses. With every new drug introduced there is likely to be another uncertainty to be resolved. Without opportunity for valid comparison with other agents, which can be done only if studies are made on absolutely comparable groups of patients the uncertainty cannot be resolved unless the differences in response are so enormous that statistical treatment is superfluous.

Obviously there must be good reason to approve randomized assignment of subjects to a controlled study. Ordinarily this reason will be a situation in which the superiority of one treatment method over another has not been established. It would certainly be incumbent on investigators to explain fully to participating subjects the rationale of the study. And no one of the treatment procedures should be one which is not at least potentially superior to another.

Legal mechanisms for control of the use of human subjects in medical and other research are undoubtedly necessary. In the first place, one obviously cannot count implicitly on the ethical judgment of every individual in the country or in the world who might wish to conduct such studies. The current interest in greater control of human experimentation rose, as noted earlier, out of the revelations of the Nuremberg trials which exposed the horrendous practices carried out under orders of persons with obviously disordered minds, during the Hitler regime. It has also been noted that improprieties in the use of human subjects have not been limited to this unfortunate period in history. Furthermore there are some entirely honest differences in opinion as to what is or is not ethical in the exposure of human subjects to risk, and no one person should have the right to determine what is ethically justified. The public has a right to know that there are legal safeguards to its interests and that they are being exercised.

On the other side of the coin there is, however, the obligation on the part of government at all levels to avoid the imposition of barriers through red tape and through unrealistic fears of injury through improbable invasion of privacy that medical research is shackled. Furthermore sectarian religious positions should not be allowed to hamper progress. The fact that one or a few religious sects consider the product of conception to have the rights of a human individual from the moment of fertilization of an ovum by a sperm, for example, does not justify enforcing behavior based on such a dogma upon the entire remainder of society which does not hold such views. There is always the danger when laws or regulations of administrative agencies are laid down or interpreted for execution that political pressure groups will exert undue influence. Genuine ethical concerns may be lost in the shuffle. Society has a great stake in the progress of medical science. The people of the U.S., for example, would not be spending this year about 8 percent of the nation's gross national product on the total health enterprise if health were not considered to have a very high priority. Only a very small percentage of that total sum of money is spent on medical research but the returns on the small fraction have been very great in the past and promise to be equally great in the future–if insuperable impediments to progress are not imposed.

The law regarding the use of human subjects should not be written or administered in such ways as to impose such impediments. In oversimplified summary: Society needs legal protection against abuses. It will suffer greatly if paranoid fears or sectarian bias are allowed to dominate and impede progress.

REFERENCES

1. Hirsh, Bernard D.: The medicolegal framework for clinical research in medicine. *New Dimensions in Legal and Ethical Concepts for Human Research. Annals of NYAS, 169(2):*308-315, 1970.

2. Leake, Chauncey: The humanistic tradition in the health professions. In Visscher, M. B. (Ed.): *Humanistic Perspectives in Medical Ethics.* Buffalo, N.Y., Prometheus Books, 1973, Chap. 1, p. 7.
3. Calabresi, Guido: Reflections on medical experimentation in humans. *Ethical Aspects of Experimentation with Human Subjects.* Daedalus, Spring 1969.
4. Protection of human subjects. *Federal Register, 39:*105, Pt. II. Washington, D.C., Department of Health, Education and Welfare, 1974.
5. *New York Times,* April 30, 1974.
6. The Board of Regents' Policy on Standards and Procedures Related to the Use of Human Subjects in Research, June 8, 1973, University of Minnesota.

CHAPTER 5

On the Ethics of the Study of Products of Human Conception in Medical Research

A T THE PRESENT TIME there is probably no field of medical research in which religion, sentiment, and emotion are more completely intertwined with considerations of ethics and law than that of the employment of the products of human conception in scientific study. In any society there is a tendency for persons with strong religious and emotional biases to attempt first to convince and, if that fails, then to enforce their views of what is appropriate and ethical on the rest of society. This is happening in very obvious ways in connection with ethical attitudes and consequent extralegal and legal constraints in connection with the use of material obtained as a result of legal abortion in the United States and in many other parts of the world. In one State Legislature the Judiciary Committee of the Senate approved a bill (Minnesota Senate file #1004, 1973) reading in part: "Whoever shall use or permit the use of a living human conceptus for any type of scientific, laboratory research, or other study except to protect the life and health of such conceptus shall be guilty of a gross misdemeanor." The word "living" was defined as "including but not limited to movement, heart or respiratory activity, and the presence of electroencephalographic or cardiographic activity, and such human conceptus shall be considered living until all above signs of life shall be absent for at least twenty-four hours." The bill did not pass finally in the above form, but the final Act that was passed and is now law states "the use of a living human conceptus for research or experimentation which verifiable scientific evidence shows shall be harmless to the conceptus shall be permitted." The final Act also eliminated the provision "that all such evidence (of life) shall be absent for at least twenty-four hours."

34

In other words, the compromise bill in essence defined death simply as absence of movement, heart or respiratory activity and electrical evidence of brain or heart activity. This change would not have been made without the vigorous intervention of the Council of the State Medical Association which called the original bill "overly restrictive" and one which "it must oppose."

The Minnesota Act as finally passed, however, still raises many ethical questions as to its propriety. The fundamental ethical question raised by the so-called prolife minority is with regard to the propriety of employing any still-living cells or organs of human conceptus origin for scientific study. In considering this problem on its face, nearly the same argument could actually be used to prohibit the use of any living tissue taken surgically from any patient undergoing surgery for therapeutic reasons. For example, innumerable studies have been made on the physiology, pharmacology, biochemistry, and anatomy of segments of bowel trimmed from excess material removed during cancer surgery or in surgery for reconstruction of the bowel for other reasons. The issue of informed consent is no different in the case of an unborn fetus than it is in the case of a newborn child with atresia of the esophagus or from other defects requiring surgery. If parents are legally and ethically qualified to give consent in the latter situation, the mother should certainly be qualified to give consent in the case of an unborn nonviable fetus.

In other words, the question in this case is not really one of informed consent or the propriety of using living cells or organs from human bodies. If the question is approached honestly, it boils down to one of whether abortion is or is not ethically justified under any circumstances. Thus, it appears on sober analysis that the agitation against the use of "living" but not independently viable fetal material derived at the time of legal abortion is a smoke screen.

This is not to say that it may not be appropriate to consider separately the question of the ethics of tampering with genetics, as in experiments on cloning, or even the ethics of bringing otherwise nonviable human fetuses to an independently viable state of maturity in some artificial environment. These are separable problems from an ethical viewpoint.

From an ethical viewpoint the real problem in connection with the use of material from legal abortions would appear to be whether it is not wholly unethical to refuse to permit scientific studies on independently nonviable fetuses in order to gain information which is essential for progress in the field of developmental physiology, pharmacology, pathology, and biochemistry. In other words, one could—and the author believes, should—put the shoe on the other foot. There are innumerable problems still unsolved in the fields of fetal physiology and pharmacology that can only be solved properly by studies on human fetuses. For example, there is the problem of drug effects *in utero* depending upon knowledge of the rates of movement of drugs across placental barriers, and the sites of storage and action of drugs which do reach the fetus. The solution of these problems, especially those dealing with actions of drugs, require study on still living, but permanently nonviable, fetal material.

It is not only by attempts to put ethical concepts which place scientific studies on the human conceptus under the ban of substantive law that serious problems are arising. It is equally possible to stop scientific research utilizing human fetal material by more subtle means. All that is necessary is to refuse to fund research of such types. And this is happening. The "Protection of Human Subjects Act,"[1] as noted previously, temporarily prohibits studies on human fetal materials by law. The ban may be lifted if the Commission for the Protection of Human Subjects should so recommend. However, somewhat earlier the NIH had stopped funding research projects involving human fetuses, and the HEW had also proposed in the *Federal Register,* August 23, 1974, new rules reading that, "Vital functions of an abortus will not be artificially maintained except where the purpose of the activity is to develop new methods for enabling the abortus to survive to the point of viability; and (that) experimental procedures which would terminate the heart beat or respiration of the abortus will not be employed." Since the heart begins to beat early in embryonic life and since fetuses are not independently viable until well into the third trimester of pregnancy, virtually all physiological or pharmacological studies on the embryonic or fetal human nervous system and heart would be outlawed. The Executive Director of a national foundation, strangely enough the one devoted to the prevention of birth defects, has also stated that it would not fund studies on fetal material from legal abortions. It happens that an influential member of the governing board of that foundation is emotionally, and in his opinion obviously ethically, opposed to abortion. Thus the wax that feeds the candle of scientific research in this field is being withdrawn.

A recent case in the Massachusetts courts against four physicians who performed studies on tissue from nonviable fetuses obtained after legal abortions presents some rather remarkable features. These physicians were accused under an old and forgotten law prohibiting grave digging, of having committed actionable offenses. All of them were reported to have been suspended from their staff positions in a major Boston hospital in which the studies were carried on, until the case was settled. If the courts should decide that the use of nonviable fetal material, which would otherwise in all likelihood have been incinerated is the equivalent of the grave robbing of a century or more ago, it would mean that unless the law is repealed, no one in the State of Massachusetts would be able legally to make use of any fetal material in the future, and it would also throw into serious question the legality of the scientific use of any autopsy material. As of the time of this writing, the case is unsettled, but it is mentioned in the context of the ethical problem involved in medical research using material from human subjects, because it is illustrative of the extreme lengths to which partisans of points of view will go in dredging the archives of legal statutes to attempt to enforce conformity to their own ethical positions. It is unfortunate but true that ethical presuppositions are not subject to scientific analysis. Ethical positions always depend upon some presuppositions. In the case of the propriety of the scientific study of products of human conception it is the disparity in presuppositions between one group and another in society that brings about the clash in ethical positions.

It should be noted that private opinions and ethical attitudes toward abortion should obviously be respected. No one of those—and the present author is one—who sees no ethical problem in abortion before the state of maturity at which a fetus can survive independently, should ever attempt to enforce his or her private views on persons with differing presuppositions. Conversely, those who hold opposite views should not impede scientific progress in the fields of amniocentesis or scientific studies on nonviable fetal material on those who do not agree with them. It may be noted at this point that reliable opinion polls show that the majority of Americans approve of the U.S. Supreme Court decision on the legalization of abortion. In other words, one is dealing with an attempt on the part of a vociferous and highly emotional minority to enforce its views upon the majority. This is dangerous business in a democracy.

It is said that a bureaucracy can sometimes be so frightened by a vocal minority that it may completely ignore logic or the principles of scientific inquiry. The National Institutes of Health were set up to improve the quality of human life through medical science advance. The utility of the several Institutes is being eroded in this instance by the fear that a minority may be successful in cutting off parts or all of their sources of funds. Perhaps the blame should be placed on the vulnerability of the Congress of the United States to pressure tactics, because there is where the shoe ultimately pinches. The United States has lived through a dreadful period of exposure within the Legislative and especially the Executive branches of improper actions favoring special interests. It is not more reprehensible in principle to succumb to the lure of money for support of political campaigns than it is to succumb to the threat of special minority group reprisals in political affairs. Both are equally reprehensible. Outright bribery may be in a different category. But in a truly ethical system of government, men and women would vote their personal views and not be swayed one way or another by money or minority group pressures. This may be too idealistic a view for a real world, but since we are talking about ethics, which refer to a more ideal world, it would seem to do no harm and might do some good to expound the thesis.

REFERENCES

1. Protection of human subjects. *Federal Register, 39:*105, Pt. II. Washington, D.C., Department of Health, Education, and Welfare, May 30, 1974.

CHAPTER 6

Experiments in Genetic Engineering

THERE IS PERHAPS no area in biology or medicine in which fantasy has been allowed to roam more freely than in the field of genetic engineering. When the molecular mechanisms of heredity became known in principle, and in some extent in detail, some working scientists began to speak and to write as though they were creators of science fiction. So long as one is not burdened with any necessity to restrict one's predictions to developments for which there is some realistic prospect of translating the imaginary to the real, there is of course no limit to the length that fantasy can lead. So it has been in relation to genetic engineering. Aldous Huxley in his *Brave New World* led the way, but numerous others have put their fertile imaginations to work in the same directions.

There is a real problem for scientists when, in the public mind, science fiction becomes confused with scientific reality. One problem is that the public becomes frightened by apparitions which so far as anyone can judge today, have no possible chance of materialization. However, only the knowledgeable scientist realizes that science fiction is just that, namely fiction. There is the danger that a majority of the people might become so alarmed by the prospects of tampering with the genetic apparatus that they might go so far as to outlaw studies of sorts which might lead eventually to practicable and safe procedures for altering human heredity or simply altering methods for replicating individuals of the genus Homo.

Of course, there are many methods known today which could alter the composition of the human genetic pool in directions which would seem to be desirable to a particular ruling establishment in any segment of human society. For example, we need no more information, in principle, to prevent reproduction on the

39

part of individuals whose characteristics we consider for some reason, good or bad, to be inferior, or to encourage reproduction by individuals whose characteristics we consider to be superior. As a matter of fact, in some countries and some states in the United States there have been laws requiring sterilization of certain types of mental defectives. We already make use of artificial insemination in the human. It is estimated that in the United States at least a million babies have been born through the intervention of artificial insemination. It takes no great imagination to see that if the public attitude, or simply the attitude of the political power structure, were such as to promote such practices, they could easily be put into effect today. Furthermore, additional scientific research might make transplantation of human ova a practicable procedure, as it is now in the case of some lower forms of life. Furthermore, additional scientific research might make it possible to harvest numerous ova from women whose genetic characteristics are considered to be most desirable for one reason or another. It might even be possible to induce embryonic development from ova by artificial parthenogenesis, thus eliminating the need for the introduction of any genes from a male line. This process would lead always to a production of female offspring, which might be attractive to the feminist movement. It would make males in human society unnecessary. Actually, all of such potential developments are within the realm of extensions to the human of processes that are known to operate successfully in other animals. However, there are great social and, therefore, ethical problems involved in decisions concerning the application or the development of appropriate methods for extension to human use. No one can predict whether or not society at large, or some segments of human society, will in the future make use of such developments.

There are some areas in the field of biomedical genetic research in which current successful preliminary applications have already raised serious questions. An example is the use of amniocentesis and the study of cells of fetal origin to determine their sex. The obvious result of such studies is the opportunity that it provides for preselection of the sex of embryos that are allowed to survive to full term. A potential, but not as yet successful, mechanism for the same objective exists in the search for chemical agents or other methods of treatment which would allow only the spermatozoa which would give rise on fertilization of an ovum to embryos of one or the other sex to survive. These actualities and potentialities have already led sociologists to study the question of what would happen to sex ratios in the population if such methods were available and widely used. Westoff and Rindfuss[1] have studied a sample of approximately 6,000 women, some with and some without children, as to their preference for the sex of their next child. They have come up with some interesting results which indicate that aside from a stated preference among nulliparous females for a first child that would be male rather than female, and an even greater preference for a female after a first male child, the studies would indicate that over the long run there would be no appreciable difference from the current situation in the percentage of male and female offspring. The only marked difference from the present situation would be in the existence of a larger number of families in which the oldest child was male, assuming that nulliparous women would utilize opportunities for choice in their first pregnancies. The latter is of course open to question because, overall, the larger fraction of women would be inclined to use technology for sex preselection in order to balance the sexes of their later offspring and would let nature take its course in the first instance.

However, the potentiality for major disruptions in the social system if preferences for one or the other sex were to result in a major deviation from equality has led to questions as to whether further research and development in these fields is ethical. It may be noted that in some cultures large numbers of male offspring are desired for economic or prestige reasons. What becomes possible might be employed in such communities with untoward and unfavorable consequences. Thus, the question of perseverance in the search for simple and reliable methods of sex pre-selection becomes open to some legitimate question in the eyes of sociologists. It would be difficult to control behavior on these scores by legal mechanisms if the discovered procedures were simple enough, as for example, treatment of spermatozoa in such a way as to permit such pre-selection. The question, therefore, arises as to whether the possible sociological consequences of successful research should

ever be allowed to determine whether the research itself is ethical
or unethical.

There are some very obviously positive results for the benefit
of society which could be obtained by employing already existing
methodology. The sociologist Amitai Etzioni[2] has presented nu-
merical data concerning the magnitude of the load on society from
the births of one type of genetic defect which can now be detected
in early pregnancy by the use of amniocentesis. He writes,

> The consequences of not using amniocentesis are easily calculated.
> Without the test, for example, roughly 57,340 to 82,690 mongoloid
> children will be born in the United States between 1970 and 1980.
> (The numbers range so widely because data on the incidences of the
> illnesses ranges widely, as do projections on future birth rates.) The
> costs to society are enormous. By itself, the care of mongoloid chil-
> dren (which many parents dump on public institutions) is estimated
> to run to $1.7 billion a year in the United States. Aside from monies,
> scarce medical resources are used up. . . . While no one in his right
> mind would dream of forcing even one woman to submit to abortion
> to save funds or medical resources, the question is whether the pub-
> lic is or is not entitled to promote, strictly through educational and
> voluntary means, consideration of the procedure? Is this so different
> from the birth control devices society promotes?
>
> Many people are unaware of the opportunities (and risks) of
> amniocentesis, and many doctors shy away from it. The time has
> surely arrived when health authorities should launch programs to in-
> form the public of the procedure and encourage its consideration by
> all prospective parents.
>
> It is time to reexamine the taboo against genetic intervention. We
> must continue to abhor forced eugenics, provide opportunities for all
> who seek genetic services to have them, and educate the public to
> the powers and shortcomings of such techniques.

By amniocentesis it is also possible to diagnose prenatally
not only Down's Syndrome (mongolism) but also other serious abnormalities. In a rational society it would seem that it would
be a kindness to products of conception, before the period of possible consciousness, to forestall the tragedies not only to the family
but to the subnormal individual himself or herself by merciful
termination of the growth process before independent viability has
been achieved. In other words, the opposition to amniocentesis is
also opposition to abortion at any stage after conception, and is

reminiscent of the opposition of similar groups to any form of contraception. The placing of strictures of a legal character upon studies of genetic characteristics of unborn products of conception by means of amniocentesis can only be looked upon as an attempt to throttle the acquisition of knowledge, which is an old story in human society. The rationalizations for it have varied through the ages, but aside from the fact that today it is proposed only to make such studies gross misdemeanors whereas 500 years ago they were capital crimes punishable by burning at the stake, the principle is the same.

There are many other ways in which genetic information can possibly be employed to improve the health status of individuals. For example, it may easily be possible by learning the character of gene deficits before birth to institute therapeutic procedures early in postnatal life which will prevent the occurrence of the somatic defect that would otherwise result from a defective gene. A case in point now under investigation is that of a neurological disorder comparable to Tay-Sachs disease (Amaurotic Idiocy) in the human, found to have a genetic basis in Siamese cats.[3] The gene defect is expressed in the absence of a particular enzyme which could be supplied. The fact that this genetically determined defect occurs in lower animals provides an opportunity for extensive study of therapeutic measures without endangering the human population.

In quite another category is the possible development of methods for removing or inserting particular genes into the molecules that are the kernels, so to speak, of genetic material. These are processes that have not yet been accomplished successfully in any higher form of life, although it must be said that so far as one knows today, there is no reason to believe that such interventions may not become practicable in the future. However, it is undoubtedly a long way in the future.

It seems almost certain that investigators who first learn how to correct genetic defects leading to serious abnormalities in the human will have strong internal and perhaps external compulsions to attempt to put their advances in knowledge to test in the human. If, for example, it became possible to alter the genetic factors leading to a high incidence of diabetes mellitus or sickle cell anemia, or some other very serious bodily disorder, it would be impossible to say categorically that early application to the human was unethical, even though there might still be many uncertainties as to other consequences of the manipulation of genetic material which would be unknown and unpredictable.

It is unlikely that any legal impediments imposed on scientists would stop basic investigation along these lines unless society were to interdict study on genetic mechanisms in any higher form of life. Despite the fact that there are many people who might be willing to see animal experimentation made illegal, particularly scientific studies involving the use of cats and dogs, it seems very unlikely that this antivivisectionist minority will have its way, and virtually impossible that the study of other higher mammals would be totally proscribed.

There is a phase other than that of physical health in the area of human genetic engineering. Some scholars are quite insistent that it is imperative to the survival of a viable social system for humanity at large that drastic measures be taken by society. In an essay at a conference on "Technology on Trial" sponsored by the Club of Rome, Mary and James Danielli[4] had this to say about the alternatives that exist:

> We are now faced with a fascinating set of alternatives. Perhaps the most likely to be adopted is inaction until a major catastrophe destroys our social system. A variant on this theme is to tinker with the more easily soluble problems, such as water and air pollution, and leave the rest to chance. Such choices mean that we shall maintain our present value system for the most part intact.
>
> There are other possibilities. One is consciously to choose one of the following policies:
>
> *Either:* accept the genetic system of man as it is, and adjust society to match man as he is;
>
> *Or:* accept the inadequacy of the genetic system of man, and develop a new social system through genetic engineering.
>
> In the former case we have no choice other than to slow down, in a radical manner, the rate of social change and innovation.
>
> In the second case we also must reduce the rate of change, and in addition we must learn both how to make value judgements about genetic engineering, and how to carry out genetic engineering. Neither of these two requirements will emerge soon.

They are not specific as to how genetic engineering could be employed to produce a new set of social values, and they are obviously not expecting miracles soon. However, James Danielli[5-8] has addressed himself on other occasions to such topics as "Artificial Synthesis of New Life Forms," "Artificial Life Synthesis and Genetic Engineering," and "Reassembly of Living Cells from Dissociated Components." Speaking of the need for human genetic engineering, Danielli[9] has said,

> No one looking down upon the earth would be likely to suppose that man is perfect. If we look at man from the point of view of his evolutionary history, we see that present-day man is, genetically, little different from man of 10,000 years ago, and indeed not vastly different from the other higher primates. From the point of view of genetics, man is a barbarian, clad in the trappings of a civilization in which he is ill at ease, and barely able to contend. It is a civilization arising from inventions made by relatively few men, and kept in being with difficulty. . . . Our social scientists pin their hopes on the possibility of improving human institutions and environments. That sufficient improvement is possible with human genetics as it is, is a most dubious proposition supported only by slender and often intangible evidence. While we must support the social scientists in their endeavors, we must perforce consider other possibilities, if civilization is to persist and advance to a modestly stable state. The other possibilities lie in genetic engineering, if they lie anywhere in the material world.
>
> This is not to say that, if social scientists and natural scientists work together, we may not do better than separately. For example, many of the hypotheses the social scientists put forward are extraordinarily difficult to test. Critical testing could be much easier if we had available many genetically identical individuals, who, placed in different environments, would give us a more reliable measurement of the plasicity of human nature. Conversely, behavioral studies may inform us which, of the attributes of man, are most in need of modification by genetic engineering.

There are, in other words, problems not strictly medical but broadly social and yet basically biological, in which genetic engineering may well become important in the future.

From an ethical viewpoint, the question undoubtedly still remains as to whether the fruits of scientific study which would make it possible to change the general character of the human race should be encouraged. It has been said that what becomes possible will almost inevitably become real. This is certainly not a generally valid principle, but many people believe it to be true. Consequently, it is likely that many people would favor the prohibition of research that would make what they consider to be undesirable practices, possible ones.

The Nobel Laureate P. B. Medawar[10] is quoted as having said, "Almost everything one can imagine possible will in fact be done, if it is at all desirable. . . ." The question always arises as to who shall decide what is desirable. Linus Pauling[11] has stated that "the principle of minimization of human suffering" is a most important practical guideline in many areas, in fact he went on to say, "I believe that almost all ethical principles . . . can be solved, although often not without effort and difficulty, by the application of this principle." It is certainly true that there could be much minimization of human suffering by the application of genetic knowledge, both of the sorts that we have today and by new knowledge that can be gained in the future. Following the Pauling principle, in other words, one should encourage research in human genetic engineering so long as it can be assured that society will be able to insist that truly humane principles are followed in determining what is desirable. Thus, one comes back to the question of how confident one may be of the integrity of human institutions. It may seem odd, but it is nevertheless true, that the ethical propriety of scientific research which might lead to capacities to control the nature of man depends upon one's view of the likelihood that humane principles will control the power structures of society. Despite the skepticism of many articulate scholars and writers, I for one believe that an optimistic view of the future of human society is a rational one because if one looks at the span of human history, the importance of the worth of the individual has not diminished, rather it has increased. Granted, there are numerous exceptions to such a rule, and there have been ups and downs in the journey. Certainly, however, the abolition of human slavery and the general lip service at least to democratic principles, even when in reality they do not fully exist, are evidences of vast changes and I would say for the better, in the realities of human condition. It is easy to be pessimistic in the light of short-term events, but the more valid criteria must consider the long haul.

As a scientist with a strong humanistic bias I may say that I would regret any ventures into engineering human genes before large-scale and long-time experiments have been made on lower animals. I can see potentialities for enormous miscalculations in relation to experimentation with human genetic material in the present state of our ignorance of many factors in genetics. The enormous advances that have been made in the last decade in understanding the mechanisms of heredity should not allow us to blind ourselves to the great gaps that still exist in our knowledge. For example, there is a question as to whether experimental approaches to the cultivation of human ova or other cells of human origin in an attempt to devise methods of promoting development to various stages under artificial conditions are wise, even if ethical, before large-scale studies have been made on lower forms. The same is true of studies on the use of cloning. There is, however, also a question as to whether such studies are in good taste. It is certainly unnecessary to employ human material for the first studies of such processes, because material from other closely related species will serve the scientific purpose of exploratory studies as well as human material would. The use of the latter stimulates wild and emotional criticism which would not be elicited, except on the part of hard-core antivivisectionists, if lower animal material were employed. In other words, unless one is dealing with processes in which species specificity is an important factor, it would seem that investigators would be discreet not to raise the level of anxiety of the public at large by allowing alarmists to cry out that biomedical researchers are exceeding the bounds of propriety, even though in fact they may not be. In other words, there may be a dimension less than that of ethics but rather related to taste or practical prudence, which must govern medical research in certain areas if it is not to acquire a bad name.

Under the quizzical title "Brave New World?" Motulsky[12] has recently explored at length the ethical issues raised by recent and current research into genetic diseases. He also deals with such immediate ethical problems as those relating to the propriety of the use of heroic measures to save the lives of grossly malformed babies at birth. As to gene therapy he warns that "gene therapy of eggs or sperm, or of gonads, with ultimate cure may never be achieved." Nevertheless he believes that "the possibilities of cloning and gene therapy . . . should be considered on (their) own merits . . . rather than by *a priori* absolute criteria." His optimistic views are summarized, "Ways must be found to deal with these issues in a manner acceptable to most human beings. Open discussions and freedom from coercion are the best guarantees for ultimate success. The ethical human brain is the highest accomplishment of biologic evolution. By harmonizing our scientific, cultural, and ethical capabilities, the potentially achievable results can place us at the threshold of a new era of better health and less human suffering."

It is not inappropriate to note that the development of science itself has played a major part in bringing about the societal changes that have made the value of the individual a more dominant leitmotiv in modern society. Science has been not only the major source of enlightenment, it has also been the wellspring for the improvement of the practical conditions of human life. Without science and technology there could be no modern industry. There could be no freedom from disease and pestilence. Without modern technology we would not have virtually universal education and literacy in the more fully developed countries, and without the latter two, we could not have any form of democracy.

There is still another quite different area of ethics in connection with genetic engineering which has very recently come to the fore. Investigators in the field of microbiology have now reported[13] that it has been shown to be possible to recombine DNA fragments from either a frog or an insect with the DNA from a bacterium, and that the recombinant DNA can replicate in a stable manner. DNA molecules are the ultimate structures determining heredity. The Committee on Recombinant DNA of the U.S. National Academy of Sciences expresses serious concern that some recombinant DNA molecules could prove to be hazardous to man and to other higher living forms. They have gone so far as to call for a voluntary moratorium on the part of investigators in this area of fundamental biology until panels of experts have evaluated the hazards involved, which include the possible production of entirely new forms of microbial disease, the proliferation of antibiotic resistant strains of disease-producing microorganisms, and also the production of carcinogenic viruses of unpredictable potentialities.

The hazards are recognized as very serious by experts elsewhere in the world. Sir John Kendrew,[14] the President of the British Association for the Advancement of Science, has called for a permanent international monitoring agency to assess the benefits and dangers of particular types of study and to draw up safety regulations for research in these areas.

It is interesting, and reassuring, that the research scientists themselves are the ones calling for extreme caution in this area of genetic engineering on ethical grounds. Their action upon recognition of a possibly disastrous result of inadequately controlled conditions for further research is a demonstration that they recognize the validity of the ethical imperative of total honesty in the scientific enterprise as expounded in an earlier chapter of this book.

Of course, there is no assurance that scientists in all countries would, or would be permitted to, follow an ethical course, because one of the hazards in recombinant DNA studies is that more effective biological warfare agents might be produced. In a world of international conflict it is political considerations rather than ethics that frequently determine behavior. Witness the addition of three additional nations to the "thermonuclear club" in recent years, and especially the first use of an atomic bomb by the United States to devastate a heavily populated area, against the advice of the more ethically sensitive persons among those who devised and constructed the monster. One would have more confidence that socially undesirable developments on the basis of scientific research and development would not occur if recent history with respect to the recklessness of national power structures with respect to protection of humanity against thermonuclear devastation had not been so dismal.

REFERENCES

1. Westhoff and Rindfuss: Sex preselection in the United States; some implications. *Science, 185:*633-636, 1974.
2. Etzioni, Amitai: Genetic fix. *New Scientist,* January 17, 1974.
3. Institute of laboratory animal resources. *NEWS, 17:* April 1974.

4. Danielli, Mary and James: The quality of life and the values of a civil society. *Quarterly Bulletin of the Center for Theoretical Biology, 5:* 1, 29-41, 1974.

5. Danielli, James: Artificial synthesis of new life forms. *Bulletin of the Atomic Scientists,* 20-24, December 1972.

6. Danielli, James: Position paper on artificial life synthesis and genetic engineering. *Quarterly Bulletin of the Center for Theoretical Biology, 6:1,* 1-12, September 1974.

7. Jeon, K. W., Lorch, I. J., and Danielli, J. F.: Reassembly of living cells from dissociated components. *Science 167:*1626-1627, 1970.

8. Danielli, James F.: Artificial life synthesis: 10^8 years of evolution in one. *Center Report (Center for the Study of Democratic Institutions) 5:*4, 1972.

9. Danielli, J. F.: The artificial synthesis of new life forms in relation to social and industrial evolution. In Ebling, F. J., and Heath, G. W. (Eds.): *The Future of Man.* New York, Academic Press, 1972, pp. 95-104.

10. Medawar, P. B.: The new biology and the future of man. Quoted in Gorney, Roderic: *UCLA Law Review, 15:*275, February 1968.

11. Pauling, Linus: Reflection on the new biology. *Ibid.* p. 270.

12. Motulsky, Arno G.: Brave new world?: Current approaches to prevention, treatment, and research of genetic diseases raise ethical issues. *Science, 185:*653-662, August 23, 1974.

13. Berg, P., Baltimore, D., Boyer, H., et al.: Potential biohazards of recombinant DNA molecules. *Science, 185:*303, 1974.

14. Kendrew, Sir John: Presidential Address, as reported by Victor Zorsa. *Washington Post,* September 11, 1974, p. A28.

CHAPTER 7

About Studies on Children

SPECIAL CONSIDERATIONS apply to the case of scientific studies on children below the age at which comprehension of the hazards and possible benefits of such studies can be expected to be possible. The informed consent of parents or guardians is obviously essential, but over and above this is ordinarily the duty of investigators themselves to refrain from proposing any obviously hazardous studies which are not clearly potentially beneficial to the subject children themselves. Furthermore the decisions regarding studies on persons who do not possess the competence to comprehend the full significance of possible hazards and therefore cannot give truly informed consent, must be made by persons other than the interested investigator. In 1967 the Federation of American Scientists appointed a special Committee on Ethical Aspects of the Use of Human Subjects in Scientific Study. In its Report[1] it said the following with regard to studies on children and other persons lacking the necessary mental competence to give meaningful consent.

> In the case of mental incompetents and in children before the age of comprehension, the greatest problems arise because of the dangers of abuse when legal guardians are involved, because of the possibility that inadequate interest may exist. When identifiable risk exists, such populations should not be made the subjects of experimental (as opposed to purely observational) study without the approval of informed persons other than the interested investigator and the legal guardian. It is essential that experts who are disinterested in the personal fortunes of the investigator himself should have the decisive voice in approving or disapproving studies entailing any such risk to the life or mental or physical health of any captive or incompetent person or groups of persons.

There are many types of study which are or can be potentially extremely valuable to particular subjects as well as to all children. As an example of the latter one may mention the testing of poliomyelitis vaccines. Certainly it was ethically proper, after adequate animal and adult human subject testing, to proceed to small and later to large scale testing on children. The benefits to children, which were only potential at the time studies were made, have proven to be so great that the principle has been vindicated.

In many types of drug testing such as for the control of juvenile epilepsy, it is quite obvious that studies on epileptic children themselves are not only indispensible but thoroughly ethical. Perhaps one might question the propriety of using placebos as controls in such studies because comparisons of a new agent for which there is reason to believe that there might be superior properties, in comparison with conventionally used therapeutic agents, could provide a useful comparison, subject to reliable statistical analysis.

It is essential to the welfare of children in general, and individual children in particular, that the limitations and the benefits of new therapeutic and preventive measures and agents applicable to such children be scientifically evaluated. Any such first use is obviously research and should be subject to more control than the judgment of an individual investigator, even if the latter is the young patient's personal physician.

It is important to note that there are differences in responses to drugs between the young and human adults. Mirkin[2] has summarized data showing that in the newborn among a list of various types of drugs approximately half are more toxic in the newborn than in adults, while in another group the reverse is true. Lockhart[3] has listed eight basic reasons for the differences in responses to drugs as between children and adults. The failure to appreciate the differences in reactions to elevated oxygen concentrations in the air breathed, as between newborns and adults was responsible for much misfortune to premature babies in the occurrence of retinopathy of retrolental fibroplasia.[4]

Although it seems indisputable that scientific studies in therapeutic fields of special importance of children are ethical when the particular child stands to benefit in some tangible way, it should not be supposed that all types of useful and probably necessary studies on children fall into such a clear-cut category. An illustrative example might be the case of the analysis of the pathogenesis of hyaline membrane disease of the newborn. There is no doubt that better understanding of the pathophysiology in this disease would be beneficial to future victims of the disease, but there can be serious question as to whether such a study would have more than a remote chance of improving the likelihood of survival of those infants on whom the studies were made. The humane physician attempting to deal with attempts to save the life of a newborn must act under more severe restraints as to risks that may ethically be taken in connection with studies of the disease mechanism than he would if he were not dealing with such a desperate illness. Yet for the welfare of infants yet unborn who will unquestionably benefit from increased knowledge about the disease, there is a necessity for ethical investigative physicians to attempt to clarify the causes and the mechanism of the disorder in order to be able to improve future management, if the procedures are innocuous in themselves. This type of situation is mentioned in order to illustrate the seriousness of the dilemma that faces physicians who are at the same time attempting to save lives hanging in the balance and learning more about how to save such lives in the future.

There is another dilemma in this type of situation. It arises from the fact that there is a large gray area of uncertainty as to what is simply medical treatment in grave emergencies, and what is medical investigation. As noted elsewhere, every intervention by a physician is really an experiment, because no two individuals excepting single ovum twins are genetically identical, but the dilemma as to calling a procedure normal practice of medicine or research becomes more troublesome the more grave the disease and the less is known about it. This is a general problem, but it is more acute in the case of children who cannot themselves give meaningful consent.

REFERENCES

1. Lasagna, L., Ritts, R., Visscher, M. B., Chairman: Report of the Special Committee on Ethical Aspects of the Use of Human Subjects in Scientific Study to the Council of the Federation of American Scientists, August 4, 1967.
2. Mirkin, B.: Influence of biological immaturity on the response to drugs. Presented at a meeting of the Section on Pediatric Pharmacology. *Am Acad Pediatr,* October 1969.
3. Lockhart, J. D.: The information gap in pediatric drug therapy. *Modern Medicine,* November 16, 1970, pp. 56-68.
4. Smith, C. A.: Use and misuse of oxygen in treatment of prematures. *Pediatrics, 33*:111, 1964.

CHAPTER 8

On Studies in Psychology and Psychiatry

*Tell me what you are looking for and I will tell you
what you will find.*

WRITING ABOUT A BIOGRAPHY of Alfred Binet, who was the codeveloper of the Binet-Simon intelligence scale, Tuddenham[2] has recently warned that "the zealots of 'informed consent' as applied to psychological research might well ponder Binet on the distortion in subjects' performance . . . caused by knowing the experimenter's purpose."

It seems obvious that many types of psychological research would be greatly hampered and some entirely vitiated by a full disclosure of the purposes and precise methodology of the study. Fully informed subjects would not have been able to participate effectively, for example, in some behavioral studies of obedience, which have recently resulted in a good deal of public and professional criticism. Questions arise as to whether uninformed subjects may not be harmed simply by having followed instructions which they were falsely told would bring great pain and perhaps bodily harm to others in the course of the studies. Defenders of such research protocols argue that adequate "debriefing" can obviate danger of psychological harm and that it is important for society at large to know how many persons are disposed to follow orders, even when they are led to believe that another human will be harmed. It is important to learn more about tendencies toward blind obedience in a world in which human slaughter is practiced with public sanction when it is called warfare, and in which only a few years ago deliberate genocide was practiced on a large scale by persons simply following orders from a higher command in one supposedly civilized country, and is undoubtedly still going on in some countries today. Sometimes it is not racial genocide that is practiced. Political views also can be made the basis of decisions to exterminate particular groups.

The American Psychological Association has published the report of an ad hoc committee on ethical standards in psychological research,[3] in which a set of "ten commandments," called The Ethical Principles, approved by the Association are presented. Extensive comment accompanies the report, discussing the ethical dilemmas that face behavioral research workers. Most interesting from the point of view of the matter of fully informed consent of the subjects are the first, third and fourth of the Principles. They read:

1. In planning a study the investigator has the personal responsibility to make a careful evaluation of its ethical acceptability, taking into account these Principles for research with human beings. To the extent that this appraisal, weighing scientific and humane values, suggests a deviation from any Principle, the investigator incurs an increasingly serious obligation to seek ethical advice and to observe more stringent safeguards to protect the rights of the human research participant.

2. Ethical practice requires the investigator to inform the participant of all features of the research that reasonably might be expected to influence willingness to participate and to explain all other aspects of the research about which the participant inquires. Failure to make full disclosure gives added emphasis to the investigator's responsibility to protect the welfare and dignity of the research participant.

3. Openness and honesty are essential characteristics of the relationship between investigator and research participant. When the methodological requirements of a study necessitate concealment or deception, the investigator is required to ensure the participant's understanding of the reasons for this action and to restore the quality of the relationship with the investigator.

It is apparent that the Association is straddling the fence with respect to full disclosure. This is not surprising, nor unprincipled, because society has a stake in the acquisition of knowledge about human psychology.

Psychologists are also concerned about the uses to which research results may be put. In the above-mentioned report the hazards of improper sponsorship and improper restrictions on publication are dealt with. The relevant discussion is as follows:

> One group of issues that arise from the political-economic-social context of research relates to the sponsorship of research. Although such traditional sponsors as universities and hospitals continue to support research, other agencies have entered the picture: a dozen departments of the federal and even state governments, big business, political parties, and the communications media. It is understandable that these agencies and organizations support research in whole or in part as one means of furthering their institutional aims: To make peace or war, to increase profits, to appeal to the masses, to educate the citizenry or socialize its members or to elect a president. Every one of these goals (even that of socializing the individual) is potentially objectionable. May an ethically responsible research psychologist accept support from an organization with personally objectionable aims if he believes the research will have other beneficial effects?
>
> Sometimes the sponsors of research offer support with strings attached, not allowing publication or permitting it only if the results come out a certain way. Given a scientific commitment to the free dissemination of knowledge, is it ethically permissible for an investigator to accept research funds under such restrictions?
>
> It is apparent that psychologists and social anthropologists deal with many potentially explosive public problems and that many types of ethical problems arise in connection with their participation in such studies.
>
> Psychologists also deal with ethical problems in the medical sphere. Reactions to pain, cardiac conditioning or induction of high levels of physical or mental fatigue are examples. Aversive therapy in conditioning studies and studies of drug effects upon behavioral performance are other types of research with important implications. In their comment regarding drug studies they say there is "a real dilemma because complete honesty about drug tests means that the active medication must overcome a very strong placebo effect prior to being classified as active—thus, honesty to the experimental participant about the placebo deprives us of the opportunity to distinguish the psychological from the physiological (pharmacological) effect of a drug-taking regimen.

There is considerable concern about the maintenance of confidentiality in any psychological study with human subjects. The right to privacy is one of the ten Ethical Principles of the American Psychological Association. In this they stress the need to disclose to prospective subjects, when the possibility exists that others might gain access to confidential information, that that fact should be explained to such prospective participants in a study, as part of the essential information given in connection with obtaining informed consent.

As to the performance of studies on human subjects who are mentally disabled and institutionalized for one reason or another, the Department of HEW has proposed very definite rules. In its proposed policy statement[4] it includes among those mentally disabled and institutionalized "individuals who are mentally ill, mentally retarded, emotionally disturbed or senile, regardless of their legal status or basis of institutionalization." It includes among "institutionalized mentally disabled individuals," patients in public or private mental hospitals, psychiatric patients in general hospitals, as well as those residing in halfway houses or nursing homes.

Such institutionalized mentally disabled individuals may not be made the subject of study unless "the proposed activity is related to the etiology, pathogenesis, prevention, diagnosis, or treatment of mental disability or the management, training, or rehabilitation of the mentally disabled and seeks information which cannot be obtained from subjects who are not institutionalized mentally disabled." It will be apparent that this regulation is aimed at prohibition of studies on the mentally handicapped which do not have special relevance to the particular psychiatric problems of individual patients themselves. Not only would such a rule appear to preclude the performance of studies such as those carried on in the past on vaccination against such diseases as poliomyelitis, but there is real question as to whether a control group of institutionalized mentally disabled persons with a different diagnosis could be employed to study the effects of a potentially useful therapeutic agent in a group with a type of disability which might conceivably obtain benefit from a new treatment regimen whether it be the use of a pharmacologic agent, diet, or even exercise, play or other environmental or management variable.

In addition, the proposed regulations stress, as they do in the case of prison inmates, the absence of any possible inducements to voluntary participation after informed consent on the part of the individual or a representative with legal authority to consent on behalf of the individual. The organizational review committee must ascertain that there are no undue inducements to participation involving "the earnings, living conditions, medical care, quality of food, and amenities offered to participants in the activity (that) would be better than those generally available to the mentally disabled at the institutions."

Whether such discouragements to the study of the institutionalized mentally disabled are in the public interest is, of course, a matter for society at large to decide. The regulations have obviously been written to provide protection for the individual. Whether the protection is real or imaginary will in many instances be unclear. For example, the mentally disabled obtained as much advantage from the conquest of poliomyelitis as did any other group in society. The studies at Willowbrook on mentally retarded children, which led to better mechanisms of control of infectious hepatitis which was endemic in the institution, had nothing whatever to do with the reasons for the children being placed in the institution, although it might be slipped under the guidelines under the rubric of "management." But it could hardly be said that such information could not have been obtained from subjects who were not institutionalized. However, the risk factor would have been very much greater for children in a noninstitutionalized setting, because in the institution in question virtually all inmates eventually acquired the disease when unprotected.

The moral seems to be that overprotection may actually be leading to underprotection as far as benefits to the individual are concerned.

There can be no doubt, however, that the setting up of guidelines for the ethical study of human subjects in the category of institutionalized mentally disabled individuals as well as with respect to all persons with limited freedom is a necessary development. The setting up of organizational review committees by itself will tend to improve the quality of research that is done in mental hospitals as well as to prevent outright abuses. The exercise of common sense, both at the organizational review committee level and at the HEW departmental level will be essential, however, if legitimate research studies are not to be inhibited or prevented.

The problem of distinguishing between what is research and what is called routine treatment by physicians and psychiatrists is still a vexing question. In any set of maladies as complex and as poorly understood as those encompassed under the descriptive title of mentally disabled, almost any therapeutic procedure is an experiment in any individual case. This is true regardless of whether the professional and institutional authorities in charge call it that or not. Consequently, almost every therapeutic regimen could without any stretch of the imagination be called research on human subjects, especially when the results of treatment may be subjected to statistical analysis and evaluation. This author's own view on the matter is that any development which can improve the prospects for success in the management of mental illness under the conditions under which the mentally disabled have to live, is desirable and is ethical if performed with the informed consent of parents, legal guardians, or the patients themselves if their mental state is such as to permit comprehension. Any unnecessary restraints beyond this point and beyond subjecting experimental protocol to independent expert control so as to improve the scientific caliber of studies that may be performed, will be counterproductive both to the individual and to society.

REFERENCES

1. Tuddenham, Read D.: Fame and oblivion. *Science, 183:*1071-1072, 1974.
2. Tuddenham, Read D.: *Ibid.*
3. *Ethical Principles in the Conduct of Research with Human Participants.* Washington, D.C., American Psychological Association.
4. Protection of human subjects. Proposed policy statement, Department of Health, Education and Welfare. *Federal Register, 39:*30655-30656, August 23, 1974.

CHAPTER 9

Medical Research in Prisons

"Cheaper Than Chimpanzees"

THE ABOVE SUBTITLE to an analysis of the ethics of the use of prison inmates in medical research reveals the skepticism with which many persons view the practice. In her book, in a chapter under the above title, Jessica Mitford[1] details many instances of questionable procedures in relation to the control of human experimentation in prison populations, but she fails to distinguish clearly between some quite obviously improper practices and some undoubtedly ethical and legitimate studies that have been made.

Unfortunately, there is a blurring of both definition of and responsibility for certain types of "experiments" and presumed "disciplinary" procedures in prisons at the present time. Jerome Dial[2] has reported at length on the "behavioral modification" methods now in use in some federal prisons. Brainwashing techniques are camouflaged as disciplinary actions, although in reality they are purely experimental in character. Dial says, "The worst abuses of prisoners take place in exactly those prisons where psychiatrists have the most influence." He further quotes an inmate report, "The so-called START program is designed to place all revolutionary, active convicts in isolation and (subject them to) sensory deprivation, which drives some men mad, others to suicide and suicide attempts, and the ruin of the physical health of others. Prisoners are being transferred to this super racist, Nazi-like program without any due process of law. We are truly slaves: We have no rights or say-so about our lives."

In this (START) program there is no consent whatsoever on the part of the prisoner, and there can be little doubt that the physicians who participate in it realize quite well that it is an experiment. As such it is human experimentation which should be guided by the canons of medical ethics rather than carried on under the guise of disciplinary action.

There is grave doubt as to whether programs such as START could withstand a test of constitutionality. Justice Brandeis[3] some years ago wrote in a dissenting opinion, "Experience should teach us to be most on our guard to protect liberty when the government's purposes are beneficent. Men born to freedom are naturally alert to repel invasion of their liberty by evil-minded rulers. The greatest dangers to liberty lurk in insidious encroachment by men of zeal, well meaning but without understanding."

It seems quite obvious that human experimentation in the realm of behavioral modification cannot be justified as to its ethics simply by calling it part of a disciplinary procedure.

It might be considered to be beyond the scope of a discussion of ethics in medical research to enter into questions of the appropriateness of the current prison system for incarceration of persons convicted of crime. The problem of the effectiveness of deprivation of freedom as an effective means of rehabilitation certainly has features which only psychiatrists and psychologists can study effectively and should be encouraged to do so under proper conditions. The high rate of recidivism after confinement in American prisons leads one to conclude that the present system has been a dismal failure.

For reasons which will be outlined, it appears to be not inappropriate to allow fully informed prison inmates to participate voluntarily as subjects in medical research, even research on behavior modification. In the past there has undoubtedly been considerable abuse of prisoners in connection with various types of biomedical investigation including, but not limited to, the drug testing which has received the widest attention. Prisoners' rights can be and have been abused more readily than those who are not in the custody of penal officers.[4]

The U.S. Department of HEW has published a proposed set of regulations[5] to govern the recruitment of prison inmates for any biomedical research. These proposals are for the most part ones with which any humanistically inclined person would agree wholeheartedly. There are, however, certain elements which may make it impossible for studies like those at the Attica prison to be carried on. There is so great an emphasis upon prohibiting "inducements," such as improved medical care, better food, and monetary rewards, that it may become impossible to carry out entirely appropriate studies. The HEW proposals seem to ignore entirely the possible benefit to society at large and to the prison inmate in encouraging prisoners to perform ethically proper and humanly useful service, both with regard to improvement in chances for rehabilitation of a convicted criminal, and with respect to the possible societal gain from the scientific results to be obtained. The applicable sections of the HEW proposed regulations read precisely:

§46.404 Additional duties of the organizational review committee where prisoners are involved.
(a)(1) Determine that there will be no undue inducements to participation by prisoners as subjects in the activity, taking into account such factors as whether the earnings, living conditions, medical care, quality of food, and amenities offered to participants in the activity would be better than those generally available to the prisoners;
(a)(2) Determine that (i) all aspects of the activity would be appropriate for performance on nonprisoners, or (ii) the activity involves negligible risk to the subjects and is for the purpose of studying the effect of incarceration on such subjects;
(a)(4) Determine that rates of remuneration are consistent with the anticipated duration of the activity, but not in excess of that paid for other employment generally available to inmates of the facility in question.

The prohibition of studies which could not be ethically conducted on persons other than prison inmates is perfectly proper if propriety means appropriate for anyone giving informed consent, and provided it is recognized that even prison inmates deserve compensation, as would other subjects, for acceptance of periods of distress or discomfort that may be entailed, as for example, in skin transplantation studies. To refuse to compensate a person, simply because he or she is in confinement as a convicted criminal, by reasonable and decent rewards for service to society seems at best to be somewhat stupid. At worst it appears to be a disavowal of the principles on which our society is presumably based, namely that rewards are related to service to society. We have been inured in recent years to many types of repudiation of principle in high places in the United States, but this is no justification for scientists to repudiate their commitment to honesty, integrity and devotion to the common good–the greatest good for the greatest number–in their view of their ethical responsibilities. This philosophy is not unrelated to the problem of ethical proprieties in the acceptance of the participation of prisoners in medical research. Any impediments placed by government in such participation will ultimately have to stand the test of a broader ethic than that now proposed especially in the paragraph designated (a)(1) by the Department of HEW in its current proposals. Hopefully this section will be interpreted liberally or modified.

There are several types of dangers of infractions of ethical behavior that arise in connection with the use of convicts in scientific investigation. First, there is the question of whether duress of any sort is employed in obtaining volunteers. Apparent volunteers may not actually be volunteers if there are insinuations that failure to cooperate might lead to reprisals of one sort or another, or that willingness to cooperate may improve the convict's chances for more lenient treatment in the future. A second problem obviously arises in connection with compensation for participation. Small sums of money loom large in the eyes of persons who are totally destitute, and who in the American system of penal management are paid little or nothing for any other kind of service. American prisons are notorious for the niggardliness with which inmates are compensated even for socially useful services. Parenthetically it may be noted that prison officials are frequently forbidden by law to put inmates to work at tasks more rewarding than manufacturing binder twine or automobile license plates. Opposition until recently by both business and labor to allowing prisoners to get into anything like the mainstream of industrial production has been an underlying reason for such restrictions. The practice of keeping convicts nearly or quite penniless results in the hazard that prisoners may volunteer for paid experiments in which they might not otherwise be willing to participate.

The second hazard has to do with the relief of boredom which can be obtained by prisoners who volunteer for participation in medical experiments. It is, of course, hard to distinguish between

motivations that envisage some relief from the dreadful monotony
of prisoner existence and those that may be related to a genuine
desire to be of some service to society. Prisoners themselves give
both reasons for their willingness to participate even in experimental procedures that may be hazardous to their health or lives.

There are many good reasons for society to approve of the use
of prisoners in scientific research. From a pragmatic viewpoint, it
is certainly easier to control environmental circumstances, including diet, exercise and sleep routines among others, in prison populations than in the population at large. Thus under ideal conditions
more valid results can be expected from such studies. Furthermore, so long as prisoners are truly free to accept or refuse opportunities to participate in such studies, and so long as the motivation for acceptance is not a result of improprieties in the control
of prison inmates, there would seem to be no reason from an
ethical viewpoint why informed prisoner subjects should not be
permitted to participate voluntarily in otherwise appropriate scientific studies, even those presenting some risks to health. In fact,
there is reason to believe that providing opportunity for altruistic
human service may sometimes be an extremely valuable tool in the
salvation of what might otherwise be human wreckage.

There is, in other words, apparently nothing ethically wrong
about the voluntary recruitment of human subjects incarcerated
in penal institutions so long as the inducements are not improper.
The new DHEW regulations may impede such activities, if no inducements of any sort can be offered.

Experimental studies on means of personality alteration have
become important in the research field in penal institutions. These
studies involve both drugs and psychosurgery. There is a fine line
to be drawn between experiment and medical treatment in connection with the use of tranquilizing drugs in prison populations. Although this book deals with the ethics of human experimentation,
it is difficult to draw the line between what is experiment and
what might be called medical treatment. In this connection the
current flurry of intense interest in the control of use of all mood-
changing drugs is a factor of major importance. Recent legislation
aimed at the control of abuses in the use of addictive drugs in society at large has resulted in the popular view that one element in

the rehabilitation of convicted criminals should be their deprivation from all mood-changing drugs, not only the opiates, amphetamines and LSD but, of course, alcohol. Without much doubt, a sizeable fraction of the population believes that such deprivation is an important part of the punishment for crime. And, in fact it is probably true that deprivation from such drugs, especially alcohol, comes second only to deprivation from normal outlets for sexual activities in the personal hardships of incarcerated convicts.

For this reason, studies of useful psychotropic drugs on prison populations are frequently discouraged. One may properly raise the question as to whether this discouragement is in the interests of society. It can be argued very logically that society has compelling ethical reasons for attempting to learn by scientific study, under controlled conditions, how aberrant antisocial behavior patterns can be modified, in the interests of the persons involved as well as of society at large. There need not, and should not, be any deviation from the general principles of complete freedom from coercion, informed consent and freedom for the subject to withdraw from a study at any time, as well as the requirement that a disinterested and competent committee or board must approve of any proposed studies. Under such circumstances it could scarcely be argued that the study of the effects of psychotropic drugs or even psychosurgery would be unethical. The idea that to attempt to alter behavior toward more ethical patterns by drugs or by surgery is itself unethical seems to be as absurd as it would be to refuse to study the treatment of mental depression or cancer with therapeutic modalities. No one knows enough about the root causes of the alienation from society that leads people to steal, assault, rape or murder to be able to say that scientific study of methods of altering behavior might not be a boon, both to the unfortunates who exhibit such traits in their overt behavior and to the society which suffers from their exhibition. This is not to say that there is not also room for studies attempting to learn more about the environmental factors that unquestionably play major roles in promoting overt criminal behavior, and correcting the adverse factors as completely as is possible. Preventive medicine is not a substitute for therapy for sick people, even if in fact society itself was partly responsible for their sickness.

Medical investigators who have had experience with the employment of prison inmates in various types of medical research have written about their experiences. Hodges and Bean[6] have reported on eighteen years of experience of cooperation of inmates of the Iowa State Penitentiary with investigators at the University of Iowa College of Medicine in studies involving various fields from antibody responses to fat, cholesterol and vitamin metabolism from which more than eighty scientific publications have resulted. In the earlier years the arrangements were made with the permission of the Board of Control of the prison system, but after an adverse ruling by the Attorney General of the State, such work was discontinued until the Iowa State Legislature enacted a specific law permitting the use of prisoners for medical research at the university hospitals, providing that the participation of any inmate should be entirely voluntary and that such participant would actually be free to withdraw from the program at any time. Hodges and Bean go into the question of the motivation of prisoners to volunteer for research studies which they describe as "usually somewhat unpleasant and in a few instances involved distinct risks." They detail the obvious advantages, such as escape from the monotony and oppressiveness of prison routine, and the small monetary gain which is only slightly more than an inmate could earn in ordinary prison work. They also stress the more intangible features, such as a feeling of participation in an altruistic venture. Finally, they suggest that a few prison volunteers may look upon the venture, which involves transportation from one city to another, as providing a possible opportunity to escape. They indicate that over the many years, only ten have escaped and that in these instances there had been inadequate screening of prisoner applicants. All in all, they consider their experience to be highly satisfactory and one which has met every standard of ethical propriety.

Another investigator, McDonald,[7] described a single experiment involving a series of skin allografts which were eventually performed on fifty men who were accepted for the experiment, of whom only one dropped out of the program of his own accord although all were aware of their right to do so. It is interesting that the investigators presented a descriptive statement with regard to the experiment when it was proposed, to the 2,000 men in the Attica State Prison and that within three days 350 prisoners volunteered. McDonald writes that the fifty men ultimately chosen to participate became a group with what he describes as a "genuine *esprit de corps.*" They even established a name for themselves with the acronym SAGE, meaning Skingraft, Attica Group, Experiment. One cannot refrain asking the question of whether, if such activities had been available over a longer period of time and involving more individuals, the horrendous riots at that prison might perhaps not have occurred a few years later. McDonald says, "The benefits to the inmate are not being proposed as justification for experiments." As justification for any particular experiment, he is undoubtedly right. But the further question as to whether opportunities for such participation may not have very great value in the genuine rehabilitation of individuals who have flouted the legal, and one must of course hope that this means the ethical, standards of the community is still another matter. McDonald himself obviously believes that there is great merit in providing prison inmates with the advantages that the inmate himself sees in participation in medical research procedures. He says, "The inmate volunteers for certain advantages that are clear to him, and he continues because these desires are largely fulfilled. As the guidelines of human experimentation evolve, it is to be hoped that the inmates' point of view will not be ignored." This from Attica!

Not all medical writers dealing with the employment of prisoners as subjects for experimental study agree with the thesis that under present conditions in prisons the practice is ethical. Bach-y-Rita,[8] for example, cites the usual prison rules concerning censoring of mail, hampering access to lawyers, "enforced unemployment," as factors which make prisoners improperly susceptible to the lures of even small monetary compensation, relief from boredom, the hope that participation may improve chances for better treatment, or the converse, fear that refusal to participate might result in the opposite, among other factors, in making prisoners agree to participation. Bach-y-Rita urges prison physicians, especially clinical investigators, to be more active in pressing for such prison reforms as would make "informed consent" more meaningful and the use of prisoner subjects more fully in consonance with the ethical principles of the Declaration of Helsinki. In this position he is taking a stand with which any humanistically inclined person can agree. He has an especially valid point in insisting that prisoners frequently volunteer for participation in research projects in order to escape from the depressing boredom of prison existence, but it must immediately be pointed out that society at large is not likely to approve of making prisons pleasant places to be.

It remains true that research of various sorts using prison inmates, conducted properly, i.e. with due regard to ethics, can be very valuable to society and at the same time be useful to the psychological health of the subjects.

Since this is a treatment of the ethics of the matter, it is not pertinent to go into the details of studies that might be relevant, more than to state that there is a whole range of areas, from biochemistry, pharmacology, physiology and neurosurgery to psychology and psychiatry, in which important new information could be gathered in ethically proper studies, and should be in an ethical society.

REFERENCES

1. Mitford, Jessica: Kind and usual punishment. *The Prison Business*. New York, Alfred A. Knopf, 1973, p. 138.
2. Dial, Jerome: Dangers of behavior modification. *The Freeworld Times,* III, No. 1:8, January/February 1974.
3. Brandeis, J.: dissenting in *Olmstead v. United States,* 277 U.S. 438, 479 (1928).
4. *The Freeworld Times,* June 1972, p. 2.
5. Protection of human subjects (proposed policy). *Federal Register,* 39, 165:Pt. III, August 23, 1974.
6. Hodges, R. E. and Bean, W. B.: The use of prisoners for medical research. *JAMA, 202(6):*513-515, 1967.
7. McDonald, J. C.: Why prisoners volunteer to be experimental subjects. *JAMA, 202(6):*511-512, 1967.
8. Bach-y-Rita, G.: The prisoner as an experimental subject. *JAMA, 229(1):* 45-46, 1974.

CHAPTER 10

Ethics and the Development
of New Drugs

A S FREQUENTLY HAPPENS, attempts to correct defects have as side effects the creation of new problems. The passage of the Kefauver-Harris Act by the U.S. Congress undoubtedly corrected some abuses, but it also set in motion processes which have greatly impeded the development and distribution of new and effective pharmaceuticals in this country. Obviously ethical questions are raised in this connection. In many instances the Food and Drug Administration (FDA) has not given clearance for new and apparently useful drugs which have been in use for years without untoward effects in foreign countries where requirements for study before marketing are less difficult to meet. Questions as to the net overall advantage to society arise.

As Wardell[1] has pointed out, public interest organizations have not recognized that the consumer (the patient) has the greatest stake in the development of better means of treating diseases of all sorts, not simply in preventing iatrogenic disease and in keeping immediate costs to patients down. He believes that physicians have failed, as a group, to educate the public in this matter.

The FDA has a very difficult assignment. Some time ago I[2] suggested that it should rely more heavily on the advice of panels or committees of nongovernmental experts in pharmacology and medicine in its decision-making. I pointed out that unnecessary delays in approving new drugs could cost the lives or well-being of large numbers of persons who might be spared early death or disability, and that no civil servant would be subject to much criticism for the delays in approval of a new drug, while he or she would be in danger of losing his or her job if a single untoward incident resulted from an approval of a new agent. The FDA has recently begun to make more use of such external panels of experts and has begun to accept data from the foreign medical literature in its assessment of new drugs.

The ethical problems involved in new drug development and assessment are many. Some have been dealt with in connection with the ethics of the use of lower animals in toxicity testing and studies of mechanisms of action. Other aspects of the problem involve the propriety of utilizing prisoner volunteers in studying the safety of new drugs, particularly in relation to such problems as individual variability as to dose-response relationships.

There is, however, a broader consideration, namely the question of whether the FDA or some other appropriate agency should not be adequately funded specifically to promote the development and testing of new and more effective drugs. There has been a pronounced decline in interest on the part of pharmaceutical manufacturers in recent years in introducing new drugs, mainly because of the great expense in meeting FDA requirements for approval. One pharmaceutical firm owns a product patent on an agent demonstrated to be superior to others in many instances in preventing ventricular fibrillation after coronary infarction, but declined to proceed even with an application for approval for such use. Expense was cited as a reason. The same firm distributes the drug for such use in foreign countries where it is widely used. This example is given, not as a criticism of the FDA, which has now approved its use for this purpose on the application of the holder of a use patent, but as an illustration of the complexity of the problem of the introduction of useful new drugs in the U.S.

As I[3] have pointed out at greater length elsewhere, there are two sides to the coin in very strict regulatory rules to insure consumer protection in the new drug field. It has not been uncommon for an application to be required to have thousands of pages of detailed and largely incomprehensible raw data to meet stated requirements. One can hardly blame manufacturers for hesitating to risk millions of dollars on development of new drugs, especially since it is so difficult to convince a skeptical public that in order to be fiscally sound as to its total operations, the profit on the small fraction of agents tested that are ultimately found to be useful and approved for sale, must be large enough to carry the very large cost of research and development of all the agents tested that did not make the grade. If the public wants useful drugs to be available at prices that reflect actual manufacturing and distribution cost of those items, it would have to be willing to bear the costs of research and development in some other way. At the present time there is no other way.

The ethical propriety of regulation which becomes so burdensome that the pharmaceutical industry finds it uneconomic to supply the public with new curative agents because of the great cost of development to the point where FDA approval can be obtained can certainly be questioned. Without a doubt, the public needs and deserves to be protected against unscrupulous hucksters. But there is a wide range between essential protection based on the informed judgment of competent medical scientists and the meticulous red-tape types of regulations which, until very recently at least, have been enforced by the FDA in its interpretation of its responsibilities under the Kefauver-Harris Amendments.

What one is dealing with in this situation is the ethics of a possibly overzealous Congress and a regulatory agency interpreting the law. The question of what is good becomes entangled with the question of what is feasible in the real world. I suppose that no one would deny that it was good to have potentially superior drugs available for physicians' prescriptions for patients who might benefit from them. Nor would anyone deny that useless agents should be kept off the market. The real problems arise when potentially useful agents are also potentially harmful, or when there is some question as to real usefulness. Many useful agents, perhaps most, are potentially harmful, even potentially lethal, consequently no drug should be banned simply because it could do harm.

This is where judgment comes into the picture, and unfortunately it is not a judgment that anyone except knowledgeable experts can make. A problem arises from the fact that there is such a wide range in the degrees of competence among presently licensed members of the medical profession. The FDA has no mechanism for approving a drug for prescription by competent experts and banning its use by others. The pretense of omniscience thought to be essential by many licensed medical practitioners certainly does not make the matter simpler. If physicians were more modest and regularly sought advice from colleagues more expert than they are in particular areas, the problem would be eased. But unfortunately personal pride or economic factors too often stand in the way. Consequently the FDA may be justified in refusing to approve a particular drug for general distribution simply because it believes that it would likely be misused by the mine run of physicians.

The question still remains as to whether it is the function of the regulatory agency or the medical schools to remedy these defects. Aviado[4] has documented the abysmally poor record of medical schools in the U.S. with regard to instruction in basic pharmacology. The fact is that only a small percentage of medical schools offer prospective physicians adequate opportunity in their prescribed courses of training to learn the fundamentals of pharmacology. Perhaps this is the greatest moral lapse in relation to the problem of making new drugs safely available to persons (patients) who would benefit from them. The FDA certainly cannot be blamed for inadequacies in the medical science backgrounds of physicians. The medical school faculties are largely responsible, although licensing boards bear a part of the blame.

It will be apparent that there is a strong interrelationship between general medical competence and medical research in relation to the entire drug problem. The fact is that every time a physician prescribes a drug he is performing an experiment because no two persons, excepting identical (single ovum) twins are actually alike. This is why it is so necessary in any really ethical practice of medicine for a physician to be scientifically trained. The trend today appears, however, to be in the opposite direction as I[5] have pointed out more explicitly elsewhere.

Medical school faculties have not been solely responsible for what has been referred to as "an anti-intellectual movement in medicine."[6] The general malaise of the young in the years of their disillusionment over the misuses of scientific advances by the military in various countries, including our own, the breakdown of the family structure for various reasons including the population explosion, the loss of confidence in the American system of politics and especially of equal justice, these and other factors have undoubtedly triggered the so-called student revolution. Medical students have called for a more humanistically oriented experience in undergraduate medical education. There is certainly nothing wrong about a call for more humanistic ethical concern in medical education, the practice of medicine or especially in medical research. The only thing wrong about the current trend of thought is the erroneous notion that scientific knowledge and humanistic concern are incompatibles. In fact, real humanistic concern cannot be implemented in medicine without a scientific base for the practice of medicine. It is an illusion that human sympathy can substitute for scientific competence in the practice of good medicine.

Although the above thesis transcends the field of drug development, it is in this area that it has one of its most important applications.

REFERENCES

1. Wardell, W. M.: Drug development, regulation, and the practice of medicine. *JAMA, 229(11):*1457-1461, 1974.
2. Visscher, M. B.: Letters: New drugs—The tortuous road to approval. *Science 156:*313, 1967.
3. Visscher, M. B.: The two sides of the coin in the regulation of experimental medicine. *Annals of the New York Academy of Science, 169 (2):*319-329, 1970.
4. Aviado, D. M.: In *Pharmacologic Principles of Medical Practice.* Appendix A1. Baltimore, Williams and Wilkins Co., 1972, pp. 1207-1210.
5. Visscher, M. B.: The decline in emphasis on basic medical sciences in medical schools curricula. *The Physiologist, 16(1):*43-54, 1973; and Will medicine be a learned profession tomorrow? *Journal of Bell Museum of Pathology.* Publication #3, 1973; and Basic scientific education for the future of medicine. *Federation Proc. 33(9):* 1996-1998, September 1974.
6. Editorial. An anti-intellectual movement in medicine. *JAMA, 227(4):* 432-434, 1974.

CHAPTER 11

The Ethics of the Use of Lower Animals in Scientific Study

THERE IS A MINORITY of the human race who categorically deny the ethical propriety of the sacrifice of lower animal life under any conditions for the advancement of scientific knowledge. However, the numbers of these persons who call themselves antivivisectionists, and particularly their uncritical supporters, appear to be growing and consequently an analysis of the background of their positions seems to be essential. The analysis is also necessary today in view of the growing fraction of persons in the Western world who appear to have lost their bearings in ethical theory and practice.

In an earlier day in the Judeo-Christian world the authoritarian dogma that lower animals were created for the service of man provided an adequate justification for their use in scientific study. Today, however, for large segments of society the situation has changed. No documentation is needed to sustain the assertion that the authority of Judeo-Christian cosmology has lost much popular ground in the last several centuries, and opinions regarding the origin and the place of man and other animals in the universe have also changed. The explosion in scientific knowledge and particularly the popularization of crucial aspects of it in relation to both cosmology and the evolution of life on our planet have resulted in a major revolution in background thinking about literalism in interpretation of ancient stories about creation which were once accepted by most of the literates and illiterates alike in the Western World as authoritative and reliable accounts. Today, for example, after everyone with a television set has seen men walking on the moon, and with spaceships sending us information about the other planets in our solar system, it has become difficult or impossible for anyone with much logical capacity to believe that the planet Earth is the center of the universe. In connection with the origin of the human race, comparable great shifts in views have occurred. Even a quarter of a century ago, although the statistical facts about overall genetic inheritance were known, the genetic coding mechanism was still a mystery. Today it is difficult for anyone who puts trust in observation and logic to doubt that the same basic mechanisms which control human heredity were in operation billions of years ago in less elaborate form controlling morphogenesis in primitive organisms. The kinship of man with other forms of life can be doubted only by those who reject the methods of science as useful and ultimately reliable in unravelling the secrets of nature.

The superior place of the genus *Homo sapiens* in the hierarchy of living things has not been altered, however. Scientific study of man in comparison with other, presumably earlier, forms of animal life has shown that the mutations which produced a brain with a neocortex capable of verbal communication, projective and abstract logic and other attributes not found in other animals, provides a basis for a view which still puts man at the pinnacle of evolution of animal life on earth.

The problem of man today is how to survive healthily on this planet. It has been that problem in different forms and contexts since the first examples of the genus Homo appeared. But the problem today has a new dimension, introduced by the rise of science and technology. The greatest problems are perhaps those of how to feed and otherwise care for an exploding population, how to limit that population, and especially how to prevent the destruction of the human race, and perhaps all life on the planet, by thermonuclear war. But the prevention and cure of disease are also prime desiderata. Scientific study, including study of living lower animals has been and will be indispensible to human survival and happiness. Even to solve the problems of overpopulation, animal experimentation has been and still is of prime importance. Therefore, clarifying a consensus concerning the ethics of animal experimentation is an important issue.

Man has, by virtue of his superior capacity for abstract and projective logic, a chance to do something about molding his environment and controlling his own behavior in rational ways. He can consider what he ought to do. Ethics is obviously that aspect of mental activity which deals with what individuals and societies at large think that they ought to do.

What people think they ought to do depends, of course, on value systems. This is where controversy enters. A person who starts, as for example Albert Schweitzer[1] did, with a value system that begins by asserting the theoretical equivalence of value of all life, from the protista to man, and giving to the life of a mosquito or a daisy the same absolute value as to the life of a human, is bound to encounter a hard time in his logic. Schweitzer did. He spoke feelingly about never thoughtlessly crushing a flower or an earthworm, but he always ended up justifying the act of crushing countless plants and animals to meet a real human need, provided that one always cut a field of grain, for example, with a conscious sense of remorse that it had to be done. Likewise in his expressions about the sacrifice of lower animal life for medical research, he recognized the ethical propriety of such sacrifice but labored the need for conscious recognition that in each instance a judgment should be made. His exact words were, "Those who carry out scientific experiments with animals, in order to apply the knowledge gained to the alleviation of human ills, should never reassure themselves with the generality that their cruel acts serve a useful purpose. In each individual case they must ask themselves whether there is a real necessity for imposing such a sacrifice upon a living creature. They must try to reduce the suffering insofar as they are able."[2]

Schweitzer was a very complex personality who combined a broad philosophic grasp of the realities of the natural world with a rigid personal ethic which grew out of his contemplation of the consequences of the "universal will to live" ideas of earlier philosophers. Furthermore, he recognized the dilemma in which he found himself, as is evident when he wrote, "The world is a ghastly drama of will to live divided against itself. One existence makes its way at the cost of another; one destroys the other. One will to live merely exerts its will against the other, and has no knowledge of it. But in me the will to live has come to know about other wills to live. There is in it a yearning to arrive at unity with itself, to become universal."[3]

The philosophy of reverence for life became an overriding phil-

osophic passion for Schweitzer in his later life, but his ideas about
it began to appear as early as 1919. In a sermon he gave on February 23 of that year he expressed his conviction as to its great im-
port for man while he detailed–with sorrow it would appear–the
enormous gap between the facts of life in nature and his ideal. He
said,

> Reverence for life and sympathy with other lives is of supreme
> importance for this world of ours. Nature knows no similar reverence
> for life. It produces life a thousandfold in the most meaningful way
> and destroys it a thousandfold in the most meaningless way. In ev-
> ery stage of life, right up to the level of man, terrible ignorance lies
> over all creatures. They have the will to live but no capacity for
> compassion toward other creatures. They cannot feel what happens
> inside others. They suffer but have no compassion. The great strug-
> gle for survival by which nature is maintained is in strange contra-
> diction with itself. Creatures live at the expense of other creatures.
> Nature permits the most horrible cruelties to be committed. It im-
> pels insects by their instincts to bore holes into other insects, to lay
> their eggs in them so that maggots may grow there and live off the
> caterpillar, thus causing it a slow and painful death. Nature lets
> ants band together to attack poor little creatures and hound them to
> death. Look at the spider. How gruesome is the craft that nature
> taught it!
>
> Nature looks beautiful and marvelous when you view it from the
> outside. But when you read its pages like a book, it is horrible. And
> its cruelty is so senseless! The most precious form of life is sacrificed
> to the lowliest. A child breathes the germs of tuberculosis. He grows
> and flourishes but is destined to suffering and a premature death be-
> cause these lowly creatures multiply in his vital organs. How often in
> Africa have I been overcome with horror when I examined the
> blood of a patient who was suffering from sleeping sickness. Why
> did this man, his face contorted in pain, have to sit in front of me,
> groaning, "Oh, my head, my head"? Why should he have to suffer
> night after night and die a wretched death? Because there, under
> the microscope, were minute, pale corpuscles, one ten-thousandth
> of a millimeter long—not very many, sometimes such a very few
> that one had to look for hours to find them at all.[1]

Nevertheless Schweitzer was, in his way, a pragmatist. In another of his essays he wrote, "Proceeding along that way, I have
led you to this conclusion: that rational processes, properly pursued, must lead to the true ethic.

"Another commentary: What of this ethic? Is it absolute?

"Kant defines absolute ethics as that which is not concerned with whether it can be achieved. The distinction is not one of *absolute* as opposed to *relative,* but *absolute* as distinct from *practicable* in the ethical field. An absolute ethic calls for the creating of perfection in this life. It cannot be completely achieved; but that fact does not really matter. In this sense, reverence for life is an absolute ethic. It does not lay down specific rules for each possible situation. It simply tells us that we are responsible for the lives about us. It does not set either maximum or minimum limits to what we must do."[4]

Schweitzer was a gentle soul, with an unfulfilled yearning for logical consistency, who devoted his great talents to a practical exemplification of a life of service to the less fortunate. But he did not, as some appear to believe, think that moral scruples should, for example, prevent an ethical person from sacrificing the lives of animals in scientific study. In fact, although he did not develop the theme himself, the reverence for life principle can easily lead one to the logical conclusion that one has a moral duty to sacrifice life, if necessary, in scientific study, in order that the conditions of life generally can be improved.

A more pragmatic and more rationally consistent philosopher, the late John Dewey, wrote a definitive essay in 1909 on "The Ethics of Animal Experimentation." It was prepared as a reasoned argument against then impending antivivisection legislation. He wrote,

> Scientific inquiry has been the chief instrumentality in bringing men from barbarism to civilization, from darkness to light, while it has incurred, at every step, determined opposition from the powers of ignorance, misunderstanding and jealousy. It is not so long ago, as years are reckoned, that a scientist in a physical or chemical laboratory was popularly regarded as a magician engaged in unlawful pursuits, or as in impious converse with evil spirits, about whom all sorts of detrimental stories were circulated and believed. Those days are gone. Generally speaking, the value of free scientific inquiry as an instrumentality of social progress and enlightenment is acknowledged. At the same time, it is still possible, by making irrelevant emotional appeals and obscuring the real issues to galvanize into life something of the old spirit of misunderstanding, envy and dread of science. The point at issue in the subjection of animal experi-

menters to special supervision and legislation is thus deeper than at first sight appears. In principle it involves the revival of the animosity to discovery and to the application to life of the fruits of discovery which, upon the whole, has been the chief foe of human progress, it behooves every thoughtful individual to be constantly on the alert against every revival of this spirit, in whatever guise it presents itself.[5]

Modern antivivisectionists have attempted to wrap the hallowed robes of Albert Schweitzer around themselves. They have taken his "reverence for life" philosophy out of context and are using it to justify new attacks upon animal experimentation. Recently a collection of essays edited by Stanley and Roslind Godlovitch and John Harris[6] has brought together the views of some British philosophers, novelists and humane society activists, along with one botanist, all of whom develop one or another aspect of the theme that the sacrifice of sentient animal life in biological, and particularly medical research is of very questionable ethical propriety. Their points of view can be summarized, as the philosopher Patrick Corbett did in the postscript to the volume, as follows: "Our conviction, for reasons we have given, is that *we* require *now* to extend the great principles of liberty, equality and fraternity over the lives of animals. Let animal slavery join human slavery in the graveyard of the past!" These viewpoints are not unique to the British. Catherine Roberts,[7] an American biologist, published in 1971 in the *American Scholar,* the organ of the United Chapters of Phi Beta Kappa, a long article defending the viewpoint that the taking of life from any sentient lower animal should be abhorrent to the scheme of morality of any decent person. She said,

> Evolving life can therefore no longer tolerate the biological injustice of inflicting agony upon animals to ameliorate and prolong the physical existence of human lives. Brief respites from suffering and death made possible by the ruthlessness of scientists against lower life contribute nothing whatever to the spiritual ascent of mankind. Evolving life has need instead of gentle souls like Saint Francis and Gandhi to show us how to come together to live lives of nonviolence, in joy and peace with the whole of sentient creation. For the meek, strengthened and made wise in their decisions by divine sanction and their spiritual heritage, *shall* inherit the earth. The choice to abolish the sentient laboratory animal is an evolutionary inevitability and a moral imperative.

The range of the positions of the newer antivivisectionists is from advocacy of regulations which would put the onus of responsibility for proof upon the scientist in each case that important needed new knowledge could not be obtained by the use of cell or tissue cultures, or computers, or more sophisticated mathematics, to outright prohibition of the use of animals. Common sense appears to be a scarce commodity among activist opponents of the use of animals in scientific research. The generally omnivorous human race sacrifices the lives of many billions of animals yearly for food, not to mention fur, leather and feathers. In 1973 in the U.S. alone, 2.5 billion chickens were killed for food. Hundreds of millions of other species were also used for human food. There are, of course, some antivivisectionists who do not eat meat, fish or fowl, and refrain from wearing animal skins or fur. But the fraction of the human race that is consistent on such scores is small.

On strictly logical grounds it would appear that no one who condones any sacrifice of aquatic or terrestrial animal life for food or clothing has a leg to stand on in criticizing the humane sacrifice of animal life in relatively very small numbers for the control of disease. It is possible for adults, and probably for children after the nursing period, to live entirely on vegetable matter, but it is totally impossible to advance certain kinds of knowledge essential to the control or cure or amelioration of disease without the use of living animals of various sorts.

The outright antiscience, antirational small core of antivivisectionists would not be a great problem, except for the fact that they form the nucleus for the crystallization of much larger numbers of ordinary pet lovers who can be mobilized to press for extremely restrictive and unwise legislation. In an affluent society, especially one with an aging population of lonely people who frequently distrust other humans and become more attached to lower animal pets than to humanity, there is a danger that a dominating majority will one day put an end to the era of progress in medicine and the rest of biological science, out of ignorance and prejudice. How this could happen in a society devoted to carnivorous eating habits may be hard to envision, but the near success of the bill in the British Parliament aimed at hobbling their biomedical re-searchers, shows that fears on this score are not paranoid.

The relation of this issue to the safe use of human subjects for medical investigation can be made quite obvious. A new drug can-not be tested safely in man until it has been studied thoroughly in a variety of lower animals. Cell and tissue cultures are useful in analyzing some basic kinds of biochemical action, but drugs ordi-narily do not act simply on one kind of cell or tissue, nor do they necessarily act the same way on isolated cells or even organs as they do when other cell types are present in an integrated system. Drug efficacy and safety must ordinarily be tested on numerous species of animal in order to be able to make reliable transferable predictions as to their actions in man. The majority of new drugs tested first in a number of species of animals have shown reliable transferability of information to man. Therefore, the U.S. Food and Drug Administration quite properly requires extensive animal testing before it will authorize even tentative small-scale tests on man. The same rule is applied in practically all countries in which a pharmaceutical industry exists.

The thalidomide tragedy is often brought up by antivivisection-ists and their allies as an example of a case in which the toxic ef-fects on embryos in the human were not predicted by prior animal study and that therefore animal study is futile. The facts are that the animal studies on thalidomide were inadequate, and the rea-son for the inadequacy was simply that no tests for teratogenicity were made. Obviously, too few animal studies were performed. Thalidomide is therefore a prime example of the need for more, not less, preliminary study on lower animals before applications are made in human use. The experience with that drug should point up the ethical necessity of large-scale toxicity testing on ani-mals.

The same general principle applies in other types of medical re-search. No one would consider using an attenuated live virus vac-cine without extensive study on lower animal models. Likewise with innumerable other innovations, very extensive investigation has preceded any human application. This is as it should be if hu-mane ethics are to prevail. If there has been a defect in policy till recently, it is that too little rather than too much lower animal study has preceded trials on man.

An antivivisectionist today should be an anachronism. Most outright antivivisectionists are actually misanthropic zoophiles. Some of them, as already noted, are dressing up their opposition to the use of animals in scientific study with the wholly illustory claim that the use of animals in research is obsolete in an era of advanced computer technology and other powerful mathematical tools. But some of the critics of animal experimentation go on to suggest that, if empirical data are really necessary, they should be acquired by the use of human rather than subhuman subjects. Often the suggestion is made that the human experimenter himself, rather than a dog, cat, monkey or mouse, should be the subject. Actually many scientists have made themselves the first guinea pigs when scientific necessity has required the use of human subjects, but it would seem to approach the absurd, not to say the insane, to suggest seriously as some have done,[8] that human subjects be routinely employed in order to avoid the use of lower animals in scientific study for human welfare, as in drug toxicity studies in the instance cited.

More than a century ago Claude Bernard[9] summarized the problem when he said,

> Have we the right to make experiments on animals and vivisect them? As for me, I think we have this right, wholly and absolutely. It would be strange indeed if we recognized man's right to make use of animals in every walk of life, for domestic service, for food, and then forbade him to make use of them for his own instruction in one of the sciences most useful to humanity. No hesitation is possible; the science of life can be established only through experiment, and we can save living beings from death only after sacrificing others. Experiments must be made either on man or on animals. Now I think that physicians already make too many dangerous experiments on man, before carefully studying them on animals. I do not admit that it is moral to try more or less dangerous or active remedies on patients in hospitals, without first experimenting with them on dogs; for I shall prove, further on, that results obtained on animals may all be conclusive for man when we know how to experiment properly. If it is immoral, then, to make an experiment on man when it is dangerous to him, even though the result may be useful to others, it

is essentially moral to make experiments on an animal, even though painful and dangerous to him, if they may be useful to man.

REFERENCES

1. Schweitzer, Albert: *Reverence for Life,* trans. by R. H. Fuller. New York, Harper & Row, 1969, pp. 120-121.
2. Schweitzer, Albert: *The Teaching of Reverence for Life,* trans. by R. and C. Winston. New York, Holt-Rinehart-Winston, 1965, p. 48.
3. Schweitzer, Albert: *The Philosophy of Civilization,* trans. by C. T. Campion. New York, Macmillan, 1950, p. 312.
4. Clark, Henry: *The Ethical Mysticism of Albert Schweitzer.* Boston, Beacon Press, 1962, Appendix I, pp. 186-187.
5. Visscher, M. B.: In Dewey, John: Medical research and ethics. *JAMA, 199(9):*634, February 27, 1967.
6. Godlovitch, Stanley and Roslind, and Harris, John: *Animals, Men and Morals.* New York, Taplinger, 1972.
7. Roberts, Catherine: Animal experimentation and evolution. *The American Scholar,* Summer 1971.
8. Advertisement placed by United Action for Animals, Inc. *New York Times,* September 7, 1969.
9. Bernard, Claude: *Experimental Medicine,* trans. by Henry Copley Greene, U.S.A., Henry Schuman, 1949, p. 102.

CHAPTER 12

Animal Experimentation and the Law in Relation to Ethics

THE LEGAL SITUATION with respect to the use of animals in biomedical research is quite different from that for the employment of human subjects because lower animals have been treated legally as property for the most part, although a body of statutory law relating to cruelty to animals has also developed over the last century and a half. The first laws dealing with cruelty to animals concerned beasts of burden. The employment of horses in various ways, especially for motive power for streetcars before the advent of other means of propulsion, spurred on anticruelty movements in various countries.

It should be noted that the first legislation in the Western World dealing with cruelty to animals was enacted by the English Parliament in 1802. The so-called humane movement may be said to have begun in a serious way with the establishment of the British Royal Society for the Prevention of Cruelty to Animals at about that time. It happened that the rise of frequency of the use of living animals in scientific research occurred at approximately the same time.

The scientific revolution began along with the industrial revolution for reasons that are not hard to explain. The industrial revolution brought wealth and leisure to a segment of the population, and technological advance was so closely associated with scientific advance that interest in science generally grew. Leisure and wealth promoted the development of scholarship and the arts. Financial security in the leisure class encouraged persons who might otherwise have had to earn a living to devote themselves to scientific careers. Wealth allowed patronage of universities, museums, and research institutions.

Unfortunately, the rise of interest and activity in experimental medicine and other biological sciences requiring the use of living animals occurred before the discovery of general anesthetic agents. As a consequence, persons who pioneered in the study of life processes in animals were obliged to do so with unanesthetized subjects. Sir William Harvey, Reverend Stephen Hales, Claude Bernard and others, whose pioneer work set the stage for later developments in scientific medicine, made all of their studies under conditions which scientists today would shun. However, it would be difficult to justify the assertion that Harvey was unjustified in opening the chests of living animals in order to be able to grasp the heart and investigate its action. There was no sadistic element in Harvey's actions. He unquestionably produced severe pain, but his motivation was humane. He was intent upon testing a hypothesis which was to revolutionize scientific thinking concerning the functions of the heart and the blood vessels.

Ethical problems cannot be considered in a vacuum. They must be looked at in the context of their times. In Harvey's time there was no way to make observations upon the motions of the heart except by the utilization of living, conscious animals. In Harvey's time, too, society in general saw no wrong in hunting animals with bow and arrows, spears, guns, or trapping. Everyone knew that many animals suffered severe pain, sometimes for long periods of time, in such activities. Society in general, in other words, was not concerned about inflicting pain for some useful purpose or even in sport.

It would be necessary to say that the discovery of the circulation of the blood was less important to the human race than the temporary satisfactions derived from the sport of hunting in order to be able to claim that in the context of the ethos of his time Harvey perpetrated any cruelty. The same may be said for Claude Bernard, Magendie and the other scientists who performed surgical experiments before the advent of anesthesia. Nevertheless, it was due to the revulsion on the part of more sensitive souls in the early 19th century that the antivivisection movement got its start. It may well be doubted whether the antivivisection drive could have had force at that time if the discovery of useful anesthetic agents had preceded instead of followed the rise in animal experimentation.

The first statutory law which defined animal experimentation as "cruel," and therefore subject to regulation or prohibition, was the British Cruelty to Animals Act of 1876. The second country to promulgate specific statutory law providing licensure requirements for the conduct of scientific experiments on lower animals was, interestingly, Germany under Adolf Hitler in 1933. The statute signed by the latter on November 24, 1933, dealt with numerous problems in animal husbandry as well as with animal experimentation. For example it outlawed "forcible feeding of poultry by cramming" and the importation of docked horses, except that "the Reich Minister of the Interior may make exceptions in certain well-justified cases." With regard to experiments on living animals, all authority for the issuance of licenses was also vested in the Minister of the Interior, as was authority to issue legal and administrative regulations to put the law into effect.

It is one of the great ironies of the Nazi period that there was such great solicitude on the part of the leaders of the movement for lower animals and so little concern, or rather total disregard, of the welfare of humans who happened to be from racial stocks or of political persuasions which *Der Führer* and his henchmen disliked. Never has the association between zoophilia and misanthropia been more clearly shown than in Nazi Germany.

The Cruelty to Animals Act of the British Parliament in 1876 was a peculiar development in several respects. In the first place, there was an extreme lack of scientific study involving the use of lower animals in Britain at that time or before, and the horror stories which were told to motivate the Parliament to pass the Act were derived almost entirely from activities going on in other countries. The prime movers in the pressure groups were Britishers who escaped the London fog and the general unpleasantness of the British winter season by going to France, Italy and other warmer climates. An important factor in the political situation in Britain at that time was that Queen Victoria herself was convinced by the members of the nobility and the landed gentry who could afford to spend their winters in warmer climates that something had to be done to prevent the development in Britain of teaching and research procedures involving the use of lower animals about which they had learned in Italy, France and Germany. Historically, it is a fact that Victoria instructed Disraeli, her Prime Minister, to press for the passage of the Cruelty to Animals Act which was, despite its broad title, directed wholly at the use of animals in scientific study. A further historical fact in connection with the passage of this Act is that the "horrible examples" used for its justification came from studies made on the continent of Europe rather than in Britain itself and were made before the advent of general anesthesia as a practicable procedure. Of course, at that time all human surgery was also performed without the benefit of general anesthesia. It is unlikely that there could have been such a furor, even among the idle rich, over the use of experimental animals if general anesthesia had become available twenty-five years earlier.

The title of the British Act of 1876 by itself created a very unfavorable climate for research involving animals in that country, because by implication the biomedical research profession was being accused of cruelty to animals. In common parlance the infliction of pain came to be equated with cruelty. This is in spite of the fact that according to the Webster's Unabridged Dictionary, the definition of cruelty includes: "A disposition to inflict pain or suffering or to enjoy its being inflicted." The word cruel, furthermore, is defined as "disposed to inflict pain, especially in a wanton, insensate or vindictive manner: pleased by hurting others: sadistic." To accuse scientists looking for new knowledge of being "wanton" and "vindictive" or of "enjoying" such animal pain or suffering is possible only for paranoid zoophiles. The confusion between the infliction of some minimal pain and suffering on lower animals to gain humanly useful scientific information, and "cruelty" has however never been cleared up, and will not be so long as the opponents of the use of animals in scientific studies necessary for human welfare can continue to confuse the public about the distinction. The invention of the designation "vivisection" to describe in a blanket way all studies involving the use of animals was a master stroke in perpetuating the confusion. Actually, not all experiments are painful to animals, although some are. Kathleen Szasz[1] has written the most incisive statement on this score. She states:

The lumping together of all laboratory experiments conducted on animals under the gory but misleading heading *vivisection* has a very definite purpose, and any modern advertising agency using depth psychology to find the sales gimmick with the greatest public appeal would be proud to have invented it. For the innocent, or not so innocent public, the word "vivisection" conjures up the image of a white-coated Frankenstein monster cutting up a screaming, helpless animal tied to an operating table. The violent but complex emotions thus aroused turn against the scientist, and the gentle animal lover, who has never seen an animal experiment and has never bothered to find out to what extent they have contributed to the saving of human lives, blissfully indulges in fantasies whereby the vivisectionist is tied to the operating table and dissected alive, preferably by himself.

There is much room for semantic confusion still with respect to the legal problems associated with the "rights of animals." There is probably no basis in statutory law for the assertion that lower animals have legal rights in the same sense that the law gives such rights to humans. As far as the law is concerned, any actual offense against a lower animal is either an infringement upon property rights of the owner or else an offense against human morality. Animals do not have standing before any court and only other humans can complain that particular individuals have offended their sense of ethical propriety. Even law makers themselves in proposing restrictive legislation, justify it on personal sentimental grounds rather than on any more objective basis. An interesting example of this is incorporated in the speech before the U.S. Senate by Senator Humphrey,[2] recorded in the *Congressional Record,* in explaining his proposal to outlaw the use of dogs in scientific studies of toxicity of various agents by the military. He said, "Well, now, I may be a poor witness for this case, because I am prejudiced, but I had a beagle and her name was 'Lady,' and I am not about ready to serve in the U.S. Senate and let Lady's name be desecrated by the U.S. Army's testing of poisonous gases on beagle dogs. Furthermore, it is just an outright shame that the Army and the Defense Department continue this kind of inhumane practice." The proposed prohibition referred not only to studies on war gas and biological warfare agents and on lethal quantities of "radioactive materials (and poisonous chemicals)" but low level exposure as well. It is ironic that the same Senator was an ardent supporter of the Conquest of Cancer Act, and that further study on the effect of low level exposure to radionuclides is an essential part of the cancer research program.

Currently there is a new rash of Congressional interest in restrictive legislation dealing with the use of animals in certain types of scientific study. In the second session of the 93rd Congress (1974) fifteen bills sponsored by more than seventy Congressmen have been introduced into the U.S. House of Representatives dealing with the use of animals in research involving biological or chemical warfare agents by any agency in the Department of Defense. The rationale of the proponents of these bills ranges from attempts to reduce government expenditures and general antimilitary sentiments to pure zoophilic sentimentality. The sentimentalists usually limit their concern to dogs and cats.

The Humphrey Bill mentioned above passed the Senate by an overwhelming majority, amending the DOD Procurement Authorization bill for 1975, so as to prohibit the use of dogs in any research on "radioactive materials, poisonous chemical, biological or chemical warfare agents upon dogs." Actually the DOD research groups have carried out many studies on low-level exposure to radionuclides and other substances which have at least as great relevance to carcinogenesis as to any military mission. Some such experiments have been in progress for many years, and cutting them off would have resulted in irreparable loss of time for the solution of parts of the cancer problem. Other health-related problems are under study in low-level exposure to many industrially and environmentally important "poisonous chemicals." It seems odd that the Senate would appropriate $1 billion for a Cancer Crusade, and other huge sums for industrial and environmental toxicity studies, including black lung disease, silicosis, asbestosis, and other diseases due to poisonous chemicals, and ignore these things in stopping research related to them by a stroke of the pen. Sentimental attachment to pets can obviously sway the U.S. Senate in strange ways. Fortunately, the House of Representatives refused to adopt the proposed amendment.

The Abourezk-Waldie bills (S. 932 and H.R. 7328) in the 93rd

Congress are different and would prohibit the use of any warm-blooded animal, "dead or alive" in connection with secondary school biology instruction. Passage of such an Act would unquestionably be a major setback for biological science teaching and learning.

Bills proposing to completely outlaw animal experimentation in the District of Columbia, the only area over which the Congress had in earlier times recognized constitutional authority to enact such laws, have frequently been introduced into the Congress but never passed. In recent years, with broadened interpretations of its constitutional prerogatives, Congressional bills have been enacted in the U.S., controlling conditions for animal experimentation over the country as a whole in one way or another. At the present time in the United States the only explicitly applicable Federal statutes, Public Laws #89-544 and 91-579, are both laws dealing with the housing and care of animals employed in scientific study rather than with actual scientific experimentation. The only positive approach to control at the Federal level of the protocol of experiments is currently that exercised by the National Institutes of Health which derive their authority from the various Acts of Congress which give to the NIH the authority and the duty to regulate the conditions under which its funds may be disbursed. The NIH has adopted a policy requiring that each institution to which it grants funds or makes contracts involving the disbursement of funds which are employed in research involving the use of lower animals, must set up an institutional committee which must examine and approve research protocols before any such funds will be made available to it. In other words, the Federal regulations in the United States require peer review at the local institutional level as the mechanism for determining the propriety of research procedures. Individual investigators need not be individually licensed in the U.S. as they are required to be in Britain, nor is the propriety of particular procedures determined bureaucratically as it is in Britain.

British scientists have found that along with burdensome restrictions the 1876 law has in fact given them considerable relief from harassment by antivivisection cult members, because the law forbids anyone except a government inspector from gaining access to research facilities except on the invitation of the researcher. However, there can be little doubt that the great reluctance on the part of British scientists to attempt to get licenses to perform many types of experiments has impeded the development of various branches of medical science in Britain. The Nobel Laureate Lord Adrian[3] has stated that the Act of 1876 had made British investigators very "unenterprizing" with respect to investigations into central nervous system functions and behavior. English vascular surgeons came to the United States to learn the techniques because of impediments in their own country. Furthermore, the British law forbids the use of warm-blooded animals by students, including medical students, in their science studies. As a result, two things have happened. First, the majority of studies employing animals have been presented as demonstrations by an instructor on animals which have been decapitated prior to the demonstration, and second, in the better medical science teaching institutions, experiments which would in the United States be called routine student experiments are converted into nominal research exercises to study the variability of response to certain procedures. Each student obtains a license as a researcher. The latter "evasion" of the law is winked at by the Home Office which administers the law.

Statutory law in many countries, including France and Scandinavian countries as well as Britain, the United States and Germany, now deal explicitly with various aspects of the use of lower animals in scientific research. Mechanisms of control differ in the several countries, but, in general, it can be said that legislative bodies have conferred by one mechanism or another, authority to executive departments of government to assure the public that the manner of treatment of lower animals will not depend upon the whim of individual investigators. So long as laws and regulations do not inhibit the proper humane use of lower animals in scientific teaching and research, these developments are appropriate and desirable. However, the fact is that in Britain there is already a very great hampering of biological science instruction, and in the United States influential minorities are attempting to impose similar obstructions in the instructional field in the name of humanitarianism. It is only the very great interest of the American people in medical research that has till now prevented the passage of extremely restrictive measures.

An interesting sidelight on the ways in which well-intentioned people can obstruct scientific progress is found in the recent history of the Endangered Species Act of 1969 which was intended to assist in the preservation of endangered species, has become the basis for the imposition of intolerably burdensome procedures in connection with the procurement of such species of primates as the macacus rhesus, and squirrel monkeys which are not actually in danger of extinction. Animals of these species are used by the thousands in biomedical research annually in the United States. Current proposed regulations by the U.S. Department of the Interior would impose such hardships on their importation as to greatly increase their cost without advantage to society, and thereby limit the performance of scientific studies in many fields.

There is some evidence accumulating that legislatures are becoming more sophisticated in the field of lawmaking dealing with the conditions for the use of lower animals in scientific research. When the first legislation in the U.S. Congress dealing with this matter was passed as Public Law 89-544, it was called the Laboratry Animal Welfare Act of 1966. When this law was amended by Public Law 91-579, signed into law in 1970, it was designated the Animal Welfare Act of 1970. The amendments dealt very largely with the inclusion of animals used as pets or for exhibition in zoos and circuses, and did not focus exclusively on the use of animals by scientists. The unwarranted notion that improprieties in the treatment of lower animals occurred mainly in their procurement, housing, care, and use in scientific study was recognized by the Congress. It may be of interest that in the eight years of application of P.L. 89-544 only minor infractions such as those dealing with cage size for dogs and other animals, have been uncovered in any academic institution.

It is important to note that apparently well-intentioned laws, such as those designed to preserve endangered species for the future, or those aimed at protecting society from dangerous species of animals, can produce such a proliferation of governmental bureaucracy as to constitute a great financial burden on society, and set up costly, and in many instances totally useless, regulations which impede biomedical research. There is an ethical problem involved. The question deserves to be raised as to whether it is ethically proper for legislative bodies to mandate the setting up of large bureaus to make sure that, for example, among other requirements, a veterinarian's certificate of healthiness be provided for each rhesus monkey imported for medical research. Of course the question can also be raised as to whether it is ethically proper for the governmental bureaus to which assignments for setting up regulations are made, to set up rules which cost money without commensurate return to society. There is, in other words, a sphere in which economics enters into one's considerations of the ethical. To make research on the prevention of heart disease, cancer, or any other disease more expensive than necessary is a way of obstructing progress toward achievement of a generally recognized "good" for society. Are unwarranted obstructions to such achievements not obviously unethical? Laws can be unethical simply by obstructing achievement of ethical goals.

REFERENCES

1. Szasz, Kathleen: *Petishism?: Pets and Their People in the Western World* New York, Holt-Reinhart-Winston, 1968, p. 71.
2. Humphrey, Hubert H.: *Congressional Record*—Senate. June 3, 1974. (S. 9521)
3. Lord Adrian. Private Correspondence.

CHAPTER **13**

The Argument for Formal Study of Ethics by Prospective Medical Investigators

IT IS EASY TO SAY that ethical sensitivity is a quality that a person acquires *en passant* from parents, teachers, peer groups and the general environment during the growing up process. But this is too facile a way of dismissing the question of whether there might not be virtue in formal courses designed especially for future researchers in the ethics of the use of human and animal subjects in scientific investigation.

Brody[1] has marshalled arguments for the establishment of systematic instruction in ethical philosophy for all prospective physicians, including those to be involved in medical research. He does not propose that attention be focused on the views of Plato or other philosophers of the remote, or even more recent past. Rather he argues for attention to real problems of the present which may "foster a decision-making process applicable to specific cases that nevertheless embraces the broadest social, cultural, and technological implications of the action."

Ethical standards are actually not rigidly fixed or agreed upon in any society, nor can they be in our complex modern society. First, there are differences in presuppositions on which ethical propositions are based. Fixed beliefs about cosmology, cosmogenesis and the nature and place of man in the cosmos are prime examples of determining presuppositions. Others which are somewhat related are specific views about the propriety of sacrifice of lower animal life for food, or any other purpose including the advancement of knowledge. Second, there are large differences in the capacity of, as well as the opportunity for different individuals to consider ethical problems logically and in the light of verifiable facts. Furthermore there are fads and fashions in contemporary

94

thought at any particular time about all sorts of problems in the ethical sphere.

For these reasons, and others, it seems that systematized courses dealing with the whole background necessary for comprehension of ethical problems in biomedical research could provide valuable learning experiences for prospective researchers. Among such formalized learning opportunities is the all too obvious fact that the general public is skeptical today about the ability of the supposedly totally "hard-headed" scientist to consider ethical niceties. The notion, popularized by C. P. Snow that the scientific culture and the humanistic culture are two things apart, feeds the public skepticism. Furthermore there is a virtue in systematic thinking about the problems involved in the ethics of biomedical research, as in many other fields of ethics, for the prospective investigator to acquire a logically and factually defensible position in any discussions or public controversies about practical ethical behavior. Too many people are saying today that the art and the science of medicine are far apart, to allow one to ignore such views. Ideally the science and the art should be totally intertwined and ethical considerations should be involved in every decision and action. This will happen more easily if a learning experience in the whole area of medical ethics, including that of medical research, were to become an obligatory part of medical education.

Teaching medical ethics, or medical investigators' ethics, should not, of course, be simply a recital of some dogmatic dicta, nor an exposition of currently applicable law. To be relevant and meaningful the course content for such learning experience should be such as to allow a student to become at least a beginner in the philosophy of ethical matters. This is not to say that currently conventional ethical rules and currently applicable law should not receive decisive attention. They should, if only to make sure that students become thoroughly aware of them. But such awareness is not an adequate preparation for life in the real world of change. Much more is needed for any prospective member of a learned profession. If medicine were simply an artisan's trade, or medical research simply a vocation for curious pebble-pickers, knowledge of conventional rules and current laws would be sufficient. But the competent practice of medicine is much more than following rules. It involves judgmental decisions based on both scientific knowledge and humanitarian considerations. And the conduct of medical research worthy of the designation always involves innovation and must involve new ethical considerations as well.

Fortunately there are today many individuals and a growing number of institutions deeply concerned with questions of ethics in relation to medicine as a whole and the medical scientific field in particular. Society should support educational and scholarly efforts to make the two culture theory irrelevant by giving more opportunity for new generations of students to bring about functional fusion of humanistic and scientific interests and goals, and for more scholars to devote themselves to systematic study of the problems that exist.

Medical schools in the United States have in the past paid little if any formal attention to ethical problems. They have in general assumed that their products needed no special learning opportunities in this area. This age of innocence must end, if for no other reason than that the public is awakening to a need for more obvious human concern on the part of both practicing physicians and biomedical investigators. High grade point averages and aptitude scores, which are the criteria for selection of medical or graduate students, do not necessarily reflect anything about ethical awareness or sensitivity. Medical practice or research involves and requires both scientific knowledge and a thorough understanding of ethical issues and considerations as well. Research training institutions in particular cannot meet their full responsibilities to society in the future unless they provide and insure the use by students of learning opportunities in this field.

In a recent essay C. P. Snow[2] has said, "You cannot teach wisdom about human beings and you can't teach empathy, yet if empathy exists, it can be encouraged by those who have possessed it and have tried to express it in words." Snow is grudgingly hopeful that the human animal can learn something about ethical behavior from verbal exposition of its characteristics. Constructive changes in perception of what is ethical are what one might hope to achieve by making ethics a subject for rational discourse. It is perhaps fortunate that all scientific research, including medical research, requires a fairly high degree of intelligence on the part of persons who can engage in it successfully. Although highly intellectually gifted persons need not intuitively have "wisdom about human beings," there is a better chance that they might have or acquire such wisdom when given learning opportunities than would be true for some others. The fields of medicine and medical research require the highest standards of ethics and empathy because they involve the human person. This is a compelling reason for incorporating in their obligatory learning experiences exposure to ethical theory and practice.

REFERENCES

1. Brody, Howard: Teaching medical ethics: Future challenges. *JAMA, 229(2):*177-179, 1974.
2. Snow, C. P.: Human care. *JAMA, 225:*217-221, 1973.

The Nuremburg Code of Ethics in Medical Research[1]

1. The voluntary consent of the human subject is absolutely essential. This means that the person involved should have legal capacity to give consent; should be so situated as to be able to exercise free power of choice without the intervention of any element of force, fraud, deceit, duress, overreaching, or other ulterior form of constraint or coercion; and should have sufficient knowledge and comprehension of the elements of the subject matter involved as to enable him to make an understanding and enlightened decision. This latter element requires that before the acceptance of an affirmative decision by the experimental subject there should be made known to him the nature, duration, and purpose of the experiment; the method and means by which it is to be conducted; all inconveniences and hazards reasonably to be expected; and the effects upon his health or person which may possibly come from his participation in the experiment.

   The duty and responsibility for ascertaining the quality of the consent rests upon each individual who initiates, directs, or engages in the experiment. It is a personal duty and responsibility which may not be delegated to another with impunity.

2. The experiment should be such as to yield fruitful results for the good of society, unprocurable by other methods or means of study, and not random and unnecessary in nature.

3. The experiment should be so designed and based on the results of animal experimentation and a knowledge of the natural history of the disease or other problem under study that the anticipated results will justify the performance of the experiment.

4. The experiment should be so conducted as to avoid all unnecessary physical and mental suffering and injury.

5. No experiment should be conducted where there is an *a priori* reason to believe that death or disabling injury will occur; except, perhaps, in those experiments where the experimental physicians also serve as subjects.

6. The degree of risk to be taken should never exceed that determined by the humanitarian importance of the problem to be solved by the experiment.

7. Proper preparations should be made and adequate facilities provided to protect the experimental subject against even remote possibilities of injury, disability, or death.

8. The experiment should be conducted only by scientifically qualified persons. The highest degree of skill and care should be required through all stages of the experiment of those who conduct or engage in the experiment.

9. During the course of the experiment the human subject should be at liberty to bring the experiment to an end if he has reached the physical or mental state where continuation of the experiment seems to him to be impossible.

10. During the course of the experiment the scientist in charge must be prepared to terminate the experiment at any stage, if he has probable cause to believe, in the exercise of the good faith, superior skill, and careful judgment required of him, that a continuation of the experiment is likely to result in injury, disability, or death to the experimental subject.

REFERENCE

1. Report on the National Conference on the Legal Environment of Medical Science. Sponsored by the National Society for Medical Research and the University of Chicago, May 27-28, 1959, pp. 91-92.

Guide to Clinical Research—
The Declaration of Helsinki*

I T IS THE MISSION of the doctor to safeguard the health of the people. His knowledge and conscience are dedicated to the fulfillment of this mission.

The Declaration of Geneva of the World Medical Association binds the doctor with the words: "The health of my patient will be my first consideration" and the International Code of Medical Ethics declares that, "Any act or advice which could weaken physical or mental resistance of a human being may be used only in his interest."

Because it is essential that the results of laboratory experiments be applied to human beings to further scientific knowledge and to help suffering humanity, the World Medical Association has prepared the following recommendations as a guide to each doctor in clinical research. It must be stressed that the standards as drafted are only a guide to physicians all over the world. Doctors are not relieved from criminal, civil and ethical responsibilities under the laws of their own countries.

In the field of clinical research a fundamental distinction must be recognized between clinical research in which the aim is essentially therapeutic for a patient, and clinical research, the essential object of which is purely scientific and without therapeutic value to the person subjected to the research.

I. Basic Principles

Clinical research must conform to the moral and scientific principles that justify medical research and should be based on laboratory and animal experiments or other scientifically established facts.

---

* Adopted by the World Medical Association in June 1964, at the Eighteenth World Medical Assembly, as a guide to doctors engaged in clinical research.

Clinical research should be conducted only by scientifically qualified persons and under the supervision of a qualified medical man.

Clinical research cannot legitimately be carried out unless the importance of the objective is in proportion to the inherent risk to the subject.

Every clinical research project should be preceded by careful assessment of inherent risks in comparison to foreseeable benefits to the subject or to others.

Special caution should be exercised by the doctor in performing clinical research in which the personality of the subject is liable to be altered by drugs or experimental procedure.

II. Clinical Research Combined with Professional Care

In the treatment of the sick person, the doctor must be free to use a new therapeutic measure, if in his judgment it offers hope of saving life, reestablishing health, or alleviating suffering.

If at all possible, consistent with patient psychology, the doctor should obtain the patient's freely given consent after the patient has been given a full explanation. In case of legal incapacity, consent should also be procured from the legal guardian; in case of physical incapacity, the permission of the legal guardian replaces that of the patient.

The doctor can combine clinical research with professional care, the objective being the acquisition of new medical knowledge, only to the extent that clinical research is justified by its therapeutic value for the patient.

III. Nontherapeutic Clinical Research

In the purely scientific application of clinical research carried out on a human being, it is the duty of the doctor to remain the protector of the life and health of that person on whom clinical research is being carried out.

The nature, the purposes and the risk of clinical research must be explained to the subject by the doctor.

Clinical research on a human being cannot be undertaken without his free consent after he has been informed; if he is legally incompetent, the consent of the legal guardian should be procured.

The subject of clinical research should be in such a mental, physical and legal state as to be able to exercise fully his power of choice.

Consent should, as a rule, be obtained in writing. However, the responsibility for clinical research always remains with the research worker; it never falls on the subject even after consent is obtained.

The investigator must respect the right of each individual to safeguard his personal integrity, especially if the subject is in a dependent relationship to the investigator.

At any time during the course of clinical research the subject or his guardian should be free to withdraw permission for research to be continued.

The investigator or the investigating team should discontinue the research if, in his or their judgment, it may, if continued, be harmful to the individual.

Excerpts from Protection of Human Subjects

Department of Health, Education, and Welfare
Federal Register, Vol. 39, #105, pt. II,
May 30, 1974

SUBTITLE A OF TITLE 45 of the Code of Federal Regulations is amended by adding a new Part 46, as follows:

Authority: 5 U.S.C. 301.

§46.1 Applicability.

(a) The regulations in this part are applicable to all Department of Health, Education, and Welfare (DHEW) grants and contracts supporting research, development, and related activities in which human subjects are involved.

(b) The Secretary may, from time to time, determine in advance whether specific programs, methods, or procedures to which this part is applicable place subjects at risk, as defined in §46.3(b). Such determinations will be published as notices in the *Federal Register* and will be included in an appendix to this part.

§46.2 Policy.

(a) Safeguarding the rights and welfare of subjects at risk in activities supported under grants and contracts from DHEW is primarily the responsibility of the organization which receives or is accountable to DHEW for the funds awarded for the support of the activity. In order to provide for the adequate discharge of this organizational responsibility, it is the policy of DHEW that no activity involving human subjects to be supported by DHEW grants or contracts shall be undertaken unless a committee of the organization has reviewed and approved such activity, and the organization has submitted to DHEW a certification of such review and approval, in accordance with the requirements of this part.

(b) This review shall determine whether these subjects will be placed at risk, and, if risk is involved, whether:

(1) The risks to the subject are so outweighed by the sum of the benefit to the subject and the importance of the knowledge to be gained as to warrant a decision to allow the subject to accept these risks;

(2) the rights and welfare of any such subjects will be adequately protected;

(3) legally effective informed consent will be obtained by adequate and appropriate methods in accordance with the provisions of this part; and

(4) the conduct of the activity will be reviewed at timely intervals.

(c) No grant or contract involving human subjects at risk shall be made to an individual unless he is affiliated with or sponsored by an organization which can and does assume responsibility for the subjects involved.

§46.3 Definitions.

(a) "Organization" means any public or private institution or agency (including federal, state, and local government agencies).

(b) "Subject at risk" means any individual who may be exposed to the possibility of injury, including physical, psychological, or social injury, as a consequence of participation as a subject in any research, development, or related activity which departs from the application of those established and accepted methods necessary to meet his needs, or which increases the ordinary risks of daily life, including the recognized risks inherent in a chosen occupation or field of service.

(c) "Informed consent" means the knowing consent of an individual or his legally authorized representative, so situated as to be able to exercise free power of choice without undue inducement or any element of force, fraud, deceit, duress, or other form of constraint or coercion. The basic elements of information necessary to such consent include:

(1) A fair explanation of the procedures to be followed, and

their purposes, including identification of any procedures which
are experimental;

(2) a description of any attendant discomforts and risks reasonably to be expected;

(3) a description of any benefits reasonably to be expected;

(4) a disclosure of any appropriate alternative procedures
that might be advantageous for the subject;

(5) an offer to answer any inquiries concerning the procedures; and

(6) an instruction that the person is free to withdrawn his
consent and to discontinue participation in the project or activity at any time without prejudice to the subject.

§46.4 Submission of assurances.

(a) Recipients or prospective recipients of DHEW support
under a grant or contract involving subjects at risk shall provide
written assurance acceptable to DHEW that they will comply
with DHEW policy as set forth in this part. Each assurance
shall embody a statement of compliance with DHEW requirements for initial and continuing committee review of the supported activities; a set of implementing guidelines, including
identification of the committee and a description of its review
procedures; or, in the case of special assurances concerned with
single activities or projects, a report of initial findings of the
committee and of its proposed continuing review procedures.

(b) Such assurance shall be executed by an individual authorized to act for the organization and to assume on behalf of
the organization the obligations imposed by this part, and shall
be filed in such form and manner as the Secretary may require.

§46.5 Types of assurances.

(a) General assurances. A general assurance describes the
review and implementation procedures applicable to all
DHEW-supported activities conducted by an organization regardless of the number, location, or types of its components or
field activities. General assurances will be required from organizations having a significant number of concurrent DHEW-supported projects or activities involving human subjects.

§46.6 Minimum requirements for general assurances.

General assurances shall be submitted in such form and manner as the Secretary may require. The organization must include, as part of its general assurance, implementing guidelines that specifically provide for:

(a) A statement of principles which will govern the organization in the discharge of its responsibilities for protecting the rights and welfare of subjects. This may include appropriate existing codes or declarations, or statements formulated by the organization itself. It is to be understood that no such principles supersede DHEW policy or applicable law.

(b) A committee or committee structure which will conduct initial and continuing reviews in accordance with the policy outlined in §46.2. Such committee structure or committee shall meet the following requirements:

(1) The committee must be composed of not less than five persons with varying backgrounds to assure complete and adequate review of activities commonly conducted by the organization. The committee must be sufficiently qualified through the maturity, experience, and expertise of its members and diversity of its membership to insure respect for its advice and council for safeguarding the rights and welfare of human subjects. In addition to possessing the professional competence necessary to review specific activities, the committee must be able to ascertain the acceptability of proposals in terms of organizational commitments and regulations, applicable law, standards of professional conduct and practice, and community attitudes. The committee must therefore include persons whose concerns are in these areas.

(2) The committee members shall be identified to DHEW by name; earned degrees, if any; position or occupation; representative capacity; and by other pertinent indications of experience such as board certification, licenses, etc., sufficient to describe each member's chief anticipated contributions to committee deliberations. Any employment or other relationship between each member and the organization shall be identified, i.e. full-time employee, part-time employee, member of govern-

ing panel or board, paid consultant, unpaid consultant. Changes in committee membership shall be reported to DHEW in such form and at such times as the Secretary may require.

(3) No member of a committee shall be involved in either the initial or continuing review of an activity in which he has a conflicting interest, except to provide information requested by the committee.

(4) No committee shall consist entirely of persons who are officers, employees, or agents of, or are otherwise associated with the organization, apart from their membership on the committee.

(5) No committee shall consist entirely of members of a single professional group.

(6) The quorum of the committee shall be defined, but may in no event be less than a majority of the total membership duly convened to carry out the committee's responsibilities under the terms of the assurance.

(c) Procedures which the organization will follow in its initial and continuing review of proposals and activities.

(d) Procedures which the committee will follow (1) to provide advice and counsel to activity directors and investigators with regard to the committee's actions, (2) to insure prompt reporting to the committee of proposed changes in an activity and of unanticipated problems involving risk to subjects or others and (3) to insure that any such problems, including adverse reactions to biologicals, drugs, radioisotope labelled drugs, or to medical devices, are promptly reported to the DHEW.

(e) Procedures which the organization will follow to maintain an active and effective committee and to implement its recommendations.

§46.8 Evaluation and disposition of assurances.

(a) All assurances submitted in accordance with §§46.6 and 46.7 shall be evaluated by the Secretary through such officers and employees of the DHEW and such experts or consultants engaged for this purpose as he determines to be appropriate. The Secretary's evaluation shall take into consideration, among other pertinent factors, the adequacy of the proposed committee in the light of the anticipated scope of the applicant organization's activities and the types of subject populations likely to be involved, the appropriateness of the proposed initial and continuing review procedures in the light of the probable risks, and the size and complexity of the organization.

(b) On the basis of his evaluation of an assurance pursuant to paragraph (a) of this section, the Secretary shall (1) approve, (2) enter into negotiations to develop a more satisfactory assurance, or (3) disapprove. With respect to approved assurances, the Secretary may determine the period during which any particular assurance or class of assurances shall remain effective or otherwise condition or restrict his approval. With respect to negotiations, the Secretary may, pending completion of negotiations for a general assurance, require an organization otherwise eligible for such an assurance, to submit special assurances.

§46.9 Obligation to obtain informed consent; prohibition of exculpatory clauses.

Any organization proposing to place any subject at risk is obligated to obtain and document legally effective informed consent. No such informed consent, oral or written, obtained under an assurance provided pursuant to this part shall include any exculpatory language through which the subject is made to waive, or to appear to waive, any of his legal rights, including any release of the organization or its agents from liability for negligence.

§46.10 Documentation of informed consent.

The actual procedure utilized in obtaining legally effective informed consent and the basis for committee determinations that the procedures are adequate and appropriate shall be fully documented. The documentation of consent will employ one of the following three forms:

(a) Provision of a written consent document embodying all of the basic elements of informed consent. This may be read to the subject or to his legally authorized representative, but in any event he or his legally authorized representative must be given adequate opportunity to read it. This document is to be signed by the subject or his legally authorized representative. Sample copies of the consent form as approved by the committee are to be retained in its records.

(b) Provision of a "short form" written consent document indicating that the basic elements of informed consent have been presented orally to the subject or his legally authorized representative. Written summaries of what is to be said to the patient are to be approved by the committee. The short form is to be signed by the subject or his legally authorized representtive and by an auditor witness to the oral presentation and to the subject's signature. A copy of the approved summary, annotated to show any additions, is to be signed by the persons officially obtaining the consent and by the auditor witness. Sample copies of the consent form and of the summaries as approved by the committee are to be retained in its records.

(c) Modification of either of the primary procedures outlines in paragraphs (a) and (b) of this section. Granting of permission to use modified procedures imposes additional responsibility upon the review committee and the organization to establish: (1) that the risk to any subject is minimal, (2) that use of either of the primary procedures for obtaining informed consent would surely invalidate objectives of considerable immediate importance, and (3) that any reasonable alternative means for attaining these objectives would be less advantageous to the subjects. The committee's reasons for permitting the use of modified procedures must be individually and specifically documented in the minutes and in reports of committee actions to the files of the organization. All such modifications should be regularly reconsidered as a function of continuing review and as required for annual review, with documentation of reaffirmation, revision, or discontinuation, as appropriate.

§46.15 Evaluation and disposition of proposals.

(a) Notwithstanding any prior review, approval, and certification by the organization, all grant and contract proposals involving human subjects at risk submitted to the DHEW shall be evaluated by the Secretary for compliance with this part through such officers and employees of the Department and such experts or consultants engaged for this purpose as he determines to be appropriate. This evaluation may take into account, among other pertinent factors, the apparent risks to the subjects, the adequacy of protection against these risks, the potential benefits of activity to the subjects and to others, and the importance of the knowledge to be gained.

(b) Disposition. On the basis of his evaluation of an application pursuant to paragraph (a) of this section and subject to such approval or recommendation by or consultation with appropriate councils, committees, or other bodies as may be required by law, the Secretary shall (1) approve, (2) defer for further evaluation, or (3) disapprove support of the proposed activity in whole or in part. With respect to any approved grant or contract, the Secretary may impose conditions, including restrictions on the use of certain procedures, or certain subject groups, or requiring use of specified safeguards or informed consent procedures when in his judgment such conditions are necessary for the protection of human subjects.

§46.18 Organization's executive responsibility.

Specific executive functions to be conducted by the organization include policy development and promulgation and continuing indoctrination of personnel. Appropriate administrative assistance and support shall be provided for the committee's functions. Implementation of the committee's recommendations through appropriate administrative action and followup is a condition of DHEW approval of an assurance, Committee approvals, favorable actions, and recommendations are subject to review and to disapproval or further restriction by the organization officials. Committee disapprovals, restrictions, or conditions cannot be rescinded or removed except by action of a committee described in the assurance approved by DHEW.

§46.19 Organization's records; confidentiality.

(a) Copies of all documents presented or required for initial and continuing review by the organization's review committee, such as committee minutes, records of subjects' consent, transmittals on actions, instructions, and conditions resulting from committee deliberations addressed to the activity director, are to be retained by the organization, subject to the terms and conditions of grant and contract awards.

(b) Except as otherwise provided by law information in the records or possession of an organization acquired in connection with an activity covered by this part, which information refers to or can be identified with a particular subject may not be disclosed except:

(1) with the consent of the subject or his legally authorized representative

or;

(2) as may be necessary for the Secretary to carry out his responsibilities under this part.

§46.20 Reports.

Each organization with an approved assurance shall provide the Secretary with such reports and other information as the Secretary may from time to time prescribe.

§46.22 Conditions.

The Secretary may with respect to any grant or contract or any class of grants or contracts impose additional conditions prior to or at the time of any award when in his judgment such conditions are necessary for the protection of human subjects.

Index

113